Brain...Washed

Unlocking the Secrets to Cognitive Longevity and Brain Detox

Brain...Washed

Unlocking the Secrets to Cognitive Longevity and Brain
Detox

Copyright © *Levitas One*, 2024

All Rights Reserved

What are the NoMAD Plans?

Developed by Dr Ash Kapoor, the NoMAD Plans represent a transformative approach to health and wellness that combines the wisdom of ancestral practices with contemporary medical insights. The name "NoMAD" not only suggests a journey through the intricate realm of health but also stands for its foundational principles: Nutritional Optimisation, Mindful Adaptation, and Detoxification.

At the heart of NoMAD is the 6R Framework—Restore, Release, Repair, Renew, Reframe, and Represent. This methodology addresses the root causes of illness, combats chronic inflammation, and cultivates authentic vitality, guiding individuals through a transformative process.

Tailored specifically to each individual, NoMAD journeys are meticulously crafted to rebalance the body, strengthen the mind, and rejuvenate overall health. By integrating ancestral practices with cutting-edge, innovative treatments—all under strict medical oversight—NoMAD Plans offer a personalised pathway to sustainable, long-lasting well-being that resonates with your unique life circumstances.

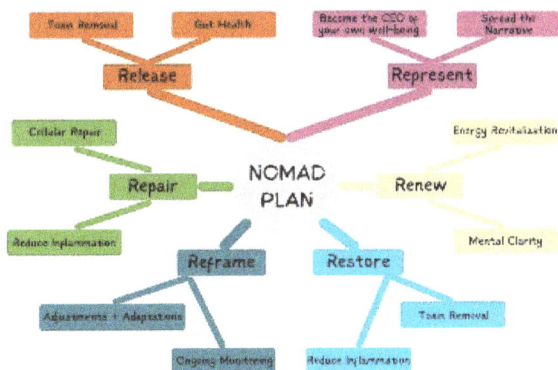

Levitas One:
"As Is In, As Is Out"

Reflecting the belief that our internal well-being is mirrored in our external environment. Founded by Dr Ash Kapoor, Levitas One serves as the vehicle for delivering NoMAD's treatment plans. It envisions a healthcare future where patients are at the centre of a fully integrated, multidisciplinary approach. Guided by Nomads 6 Rs— Restore, Release, Repair, Renew, Reframe, and Represent— Levitas One empowers self-care through personalised guidance and minimal intervention, promoting long-term health, balance, and sustainability.

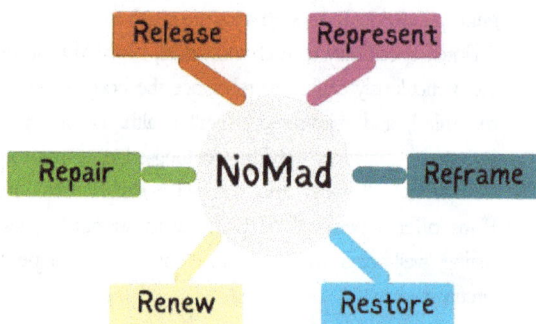

Release   Represent

Repair   NoMad   Reframe

Renew   Restore

Contents

Preface

In my journey through regenerative medicine, I have come to a profound realisation: the brain is not merely an organ that oversees cognition and thought but the master conductor of every physical process within the body. Through my years of experience, it has become evident that the brain is not separate from the rest of the body—it is intimately connected to every system, cell, and function. This insight has reshaped my understanding of health, healing, and human potential.

One of the most striking lessons I've learned is that there is no such thing as a "psychosomatic" condition in the traditional sense, where physical ailments are dismissed as "all in the mind." Instead, I have seen firsthand how thoughts, emotions, and psychological states, particularly through the limbic system—the brain's emotional centre—can directly influence **physical health**. The brain's power to regulate hormones, direct immune responses, and even accelerate healing is undeniable. What we experience mentally, we manifest physically.

As we move deeper into an era where **chronic stress**, **environmental toxins**, and modern lifestyles strain both our bodies and minds, it is critical to recognise the **brain's role** in driving health outcomes. The **brain-body connection** is not just a metaphor; it is the central axis upon which health turns. Whether through **neuroplasticity, brain detox**, or harnessing the brain's natural ability to heal, the connection between the brain and body is essential for unlocking true **regenerative health**.

In this book, I explore these themes, revealing the latest insights into **brain detoxification, biohacking**, and **cognitive longevity**, all to guide readers toward optimal brain function as the key to **physical and mental rejuvenation**. The future of healing is in the brain, and it is time to realise its full potential.

Introduction:

The Brain as the Command Centre of Life

From Survival Mode to Optimal Health

The human brain is nothing short of extraordinary. It is the command centre of everything we do, think, and feel, responsible for controlling our bodily functions, processing information, and driving our creativity, emotions, and decisions. Yet, in today's world, we often take the brain for granted, pushing it into overload through the stresses of modern life. From juggling endless to-do lists and constant digital distractions to dealing with environmental toxins and poor sleep, the brain is under constant assault.

In an ideal world, the brain would function at its peak efficiency, effortlessly handling cognitive tasks, regulating emotions, and detoxifying itself from the day's toxins. However, most of us are stuck in survival mode. The modern world's stresses—from environmental pollutants to poor nutrition, chronic inflammation, lack of sleep, and constant exposure to technology—have forced our brains into a state of crisis, where detoxification processes slow down, neuroinflammation builds, and cognitive decline begins.

This book, **Brain… Washed: Unlocking the Secrets to Cognitive Longevity and Brain Detox**, is designed to help you understand why your brain may not be functioning at its best and what you can do to reclaim its health and performance. We'll explore **ancient practices** and **modern biohacking techniques** that can optimise brain detox, boost cognitive longevity, and help your brain function like a well-tuned machine.

Why Brain Detox Is Critical

Most people understand the concept of detoxifying the body—flushing out harmful chemicals, waste, and toxins to restore health. But when it comes to the brain, **detoxification** is often overlooked.

In recent years, neuroscience has uncovered an essential process known as **brain detox**—the clearing out of toxic waste products, including **amyloid-beta proteins** and **tau tangles**, which are associated with neurodegenerative diseases like Alzheimer's.

Your brain, much like the rest of your body, produces waste as a byproduct of everyday activity. When you think, learn, or perform any mental task, your brain cells (neurons) generate waste products. This waste is meant to be cleared out regularly to keep the brain functioning at optimal levels. However, under the strain of **chronic stress**, **poor sleep**, **inflammation**, and **toxin exposure**, the brain's detox system slows down. If not addressed, this dysfunction can accelerate ageing, impair cognition, and lead to long-term neurodegenerative diseases.

Neuroscientific research has revealed that **brain detox** primarily happens during **deep sleep** via a unique waste clearance pathway known as the **glymphatic system**. During sleep, particularly **non-REM sleep**, brain cells shrink, allowing **cerebrospinal fluid (CSF)** to flow through the brain, flushing out waste. Without sufficient deep sleep, toxins, including **amyloid-beta** (which contributes to Alzheimer's), accumulate, impairing memory and cognitive function.

In the modern world, where deep, restorative sleep is often elusive due to stress, poor lifestyle choices, and technological distractions, this process becomes compromised. This is why sleep, stress management, and **lifestyle optimisation** are foundational to brain health—and where this book begins.

Modern Life: The Enemy of Brain Health

Modern life has transformed how our brains operate—**not for the better**. Consider the **information overload** we experience daily. From checking emails to scrolling through social media, switching between apps, and working on multiple projects simultaneously, our brains are constantly overstimulated. While the human brain is designed to handle complex tasks, it was never intended to manage this relentless, high-speed information environment. As a result, our brains are becoming exhausted, and cognitive fatigue sets in.

Beyond information overload, we also face environmental threats. **Toxins**—in the form of air pollutants, pesticides, heavy metals, and chemicals in processed foods—slowly build up in our systems, leading to neuroinflammation. Studies have linked **airborne pollutants** to cognitive decline, while heavy metals like **mercury** and **lead** have been implicated in the development of **Alzheimer's** and **Parkinson's disease**. The accumulation of such toxins over time can overload the brain's detox pathways, particularly when compounded by the stresses of modern living.

Then there's the role of **technology**. Devices like smartphones, laptops, and Wi-Fi emit **electromagnetic fields (EMFs)**. While these technologies bring immense convenience, they also contribute to the brain's cognitive load and may even disrupt the **blood-brain barrier**, a protective shield that prevents harmful substances from entering the brain. Chronic EMF exposure is associated with increased oxidative stress and cognitive impairments, adding to the growing list of modern stressors that hamper brain detox.

Finally, **chronic inflammation**—largely driven by poor diet, stress, and sedentary lifestyles—has become an epidemic. Inflammation is not just a bodily issue but a brain issue as well. Chronic inflammation, particularly in the **microglial cells** (the brain's immune cells), disrupts neural communication, impairs detoxification, and accelerates cognitive decline. Many researchers now consider **neuroinflammation** a primary driver of Alzheimer's disease, dementia, and other age-related cognitive issues.

The Solution: Optimising Brain Detox with Ancient Wisdom and Modern Science

The good news is that the brain has a remarkable capacity for **recovery** and **adaptation** when given the right tools. This book will explore a holistic, **multidimensional approach** to brain health, combining **ancient practices** like **Ayurveda, Traditional Chinese**

Medicine **(TCM)**, and **mindfulness** with cutting-edge **biohacking techniques** like **nootropics**, **peptide therapy**, and **NAD+ supplementation**.

For thousands of years, ancient traditions have recognised the importance of maintaining a healthy brain and nervous system. Practices like **fasting**, **herbal remedies**, and **meditation** have long been used to support brain health and detoxification. These practices, while rooted in tradition, are now backed by **modern neuroscience**, showing their effectiveness in promoting neuroplasticity, reducing inflammation, and enhancing brain detox pathways.

In parallel, **biohacking** has emerged as a way to optimise brain function using science, technology, and innovative therapies. **Nootropics** (smart supplements), **high-dose melatonin**, and **vagus nerve activation** are just a few of the tools that can be used to improve brain detoxification, reduce cognitive stress, and enhance overall mental clarity.

This book will show you how to:

- Activate the brain's natural detox pathways, including the glymphatic system.
- Use **biohacking tools** like **nootropics**, **peptides**, and **NAD+** to enhance brain health.
- Integrate **ancient practices** like **fasting**, **Ayurvedic herbs**, and **mindfulness** to support cognitive longevity.
- Manage **EMF exposure** and reduce the impact of environmental toxins on the brain.
- Improve **sleep quality** and **circadian rhythms** to optimise brain detox.
- Use **exercise** and **nutrition** to boost neuroplasticity and detoxification.

What You Will Learn in This Book

This book is divided into five sections, each addressing a different aspect of brain detox and cognitive health.

- **Chapter 1** explores the **science of brain detox**, including the mechanisms of the **glymphatic system**, the role of **neuroinflammation**, and how modern life impacts brain health. You'll learn about cutting-edge molecules like **NAD+**, **CoQ10**, and **Procaine** that play a role in protecting and regenerating brain cells.
- **Chapter two** dives into **biohacking techniques** that support brain detox, including the use of **nootropics**, **peptides**, **high-dose melatonin**, and strategies for **managing EMF exposure**. You'll also learn about **Jim Kwik's cognitive biohacks** for improving mental clarity through techniques like **monotasking**.
- **Chapter Three** integrates **ancient wisdom** with modern science, exploring how practices like **Ayurveda**, **Traditional Chinese Medicine**, and **intermittent fasting** can enhance brain detox and promote cognitive longevity.
- **Chapter Four** offers **lifestyle strategies** for long-term brain health, including optimising **sleep**, using **light therapy**, and following an **anti-inflammatory diet** to support detox pathways.
- **Chapter five** looks at **future directions** in brain detox, including the role of **wearable technologies**, **AI-driven brain health tracking**, and cutting-edge research on brain detoxification methods.

The Journey Ahead: Reclaim Your Brain Health

By the end of this book, you will have a toolkit of strategies to **reclaim your brain health**, detoxify from the harmful effects of modern life, and restore your cognitive performance. Whether you're seeking to prevent cognitive decline, recover from burnout, or simply optimise your brain for peak performance, the path to cognitive longevity begins here.

The brain may be washed—literally and figuratively—but it can also be cleansed and renewed. The strategies outlined in this book will help you **clear the mental fog**, boost your **memory and focus**, and ensure that your brain is functioning at its very best for years to come.

Welcome to your journey of **cognitive empowerment** and **brain detox**—where ancient wisdom meets modern science.

Summary: Introduction

(a) Brain as Command Centre

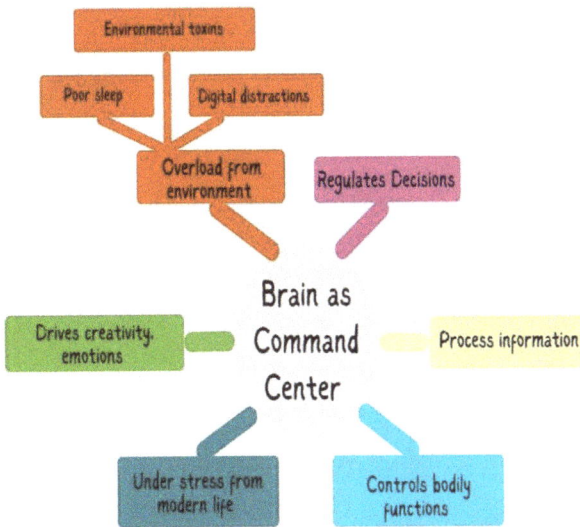

(b) Why Brain Detox is Critical?

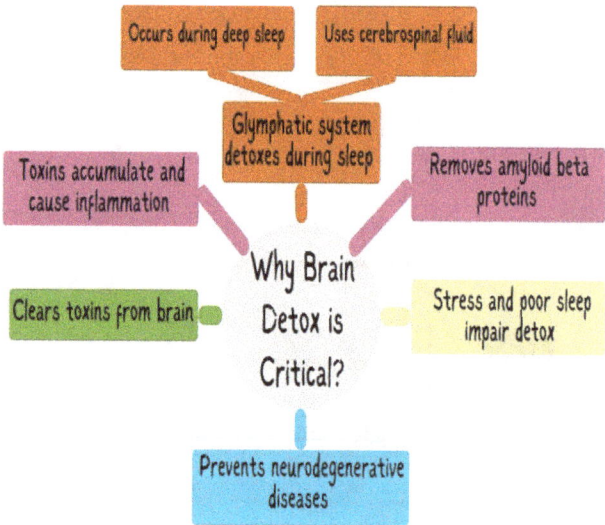

Occurs during deep sleep

Uses cerebrospinal fluid

Glymphatic system detoxes during sleep

Toxins accumulate and cause inflammation

Removes amyloid beta proteins

Why Brain Detox is Critical?

Clears toxins from brain

Stress and poor sleep impair detox

Prevents neurodegenerative diseases

Chapter One: The Glymphatic System: The Brain's Cleansing Mechanism

Understanding the Glymphatic System

The brain, unlike other organs in the body, doesn't have a traditional lymphatic system to clear waste products. For decades, neuroscientists have been puzzled about how the brain cleanses itself of metabolic waste. The answer came in the form of the **glymphatic system**, discovered in 2012 by researchers at the University of Rochester Medical Centre. This waste clearance pathway is essential for the removal of toxic byproducts like **amyloid-beta** and **tau proteins**, which are associated with neurodegenerative diseases such as Alzheimer's and Parkinson's.

The **glymphatic system** works by utilising **cerebrospinal fluid (CSF)** to flush waste products out of the brain. The system relies on the support of **astrocytes**, which are glial cells that surround blood vessels in the brain. Astrocytes create channels that allow CSF to circulate through the brain, removing toxins and waste. This system is particularly important in clearing harmful proteins like amyloid-beta, which tend to accumulate and form plaques that impair cognitive function.

The glymphatic system is most active during **deep sleep**, specifically **non-REM sleep**. During this phase, brain cells shrink by up to 60%, allowing more space for the CSF to flow through the brain, effectively washing away harmful waste products. In contrast, the glymphatic system is much less active when we are awake, highlighting the critical role of sleep in brain detoxification.

Emerging research has revealed that dysfunction in the glymphatic system contributes to the buildup of neurotoxins, which accelerates the development of neurodegenerative diseases. Poor sleep, stress, and inflammation can impair glymphatic function, leading to the accumulation of harmful proteins that damage brain cells. Understanding how the glymphatic system works and how to optimise it is crucial for maintaining cognitive health.

The Role of Sleep in Detoxification

Sleep is often considered one of the most vital processes for brain health. It is during sleep—especially **deep non-REM sleep**—that the glymphatic system operates at full capacity, removing harmful waste products that accumulate during waking hours. When we sleep, not only does the body undergo repair and regeneration, but the brain undergoes a thorough cleansing process that prepares it for optimal function the next day.

Non-REM sleep is characterised by slow brain waves, relaxed muscles, and reduced metabolic activity. During this phase, the glymphatic system becomes highly active, with CSF flowing more freely to wash away metabolic waste, including **reactive oxygen species (ROS)** and **oxidised proteins**, which build up due to daily activities. These waste products, if not removed, can lead to oxidative stress and long-term damage to neurons.

The significance of sleep in brain detoxification cannot be overstated. Studies have shown that even a single night of sleep deprivation leads to an immediate increase in **amyloid-beta** levels. Chronic sleep deprivation exacerbates this problem, increasing the risk of cognitive decline, memory loss, and neurodegenerative diseases. Adults who regularly get less than seven hours of sleep per night have a significantly higher risk of developing Alzheimer's disease compared to those who sleep adequately.

In addition to clearing amyloid-beta, the glymphatic system also removes other toxic proteins, such as **tau**, which form tangles in neurons and disrupt cellular communication. These tangles are a hallmark of **tauopathies**, a class of neurodegenerative diseases that includes Alzheimer's. Ensuring that the brain has enough time to cleanse itself of these toxins is essential for preserving cognitive function as we age.

Optimising sleep hygiene is one of the most effective ways to support brain detoxification. **Good sleep hygiene** includes maintaining a consistent sleep schedule, minimising exposure to blue light before bedtime, creating a calm and comfortable sleep environment, and addressing any underlying sleep disorders such as **sleep apnea** or **insomnia**. The use of **melatonin** and other sleep aids can be helpful for individuals struggling with poor sleep, as long as they are used under medical supervision.

The consequences of poor sleep go beyond feeling fatigued. Over time, chronic sleep deprivation can lead to reduced glymphatic activity, the accumulation of neurotoxins, and an increased risk of cognitive disorders. This is why optimising sleep is the foundation for supporting brain detox and maintaining cognitive health throughout life.

Case Study: Sleep Disorders and Cognitive Decline

Patient Profile:

- **Name:** John, age 58
- **Occupation:** Senior manager at a tech company
- **Symptoms:** Difficulty with concentration, short-term memory lapses, frequent fatigue
- **Background:** John has worked in a high-stress corporate environment for over 30 years. He regularly sleeps only 4-5 hours per night and reports waking up feeling unrefreshed. Over the past year, his cognitive performance has noticeably declined, and he's experiencing increasing difficulty recalling recent conversations or focusing during meetings. He has no previous history of neurological disease.

Clinical Findings:

- Cognitive testing reveals mild impairment in executive function and working memory.
- Polysomnography (sleep study) shows severe sleep fragmentation with decreased time in deep non-REM sleep.
- **Neuroimaging** reveals the accumulation of **amyloid-beta plaques** in the prefrontal cortex, indicating early signs of cognitive decline.
- **Lab work** shows elevated levels of **C-reactive protein (CRP)**, a marker of chronic inflammation, which may contribute to impaired brain detox.

Analysis:

John's symptoms are consistent with chronic sleep deprivation and its detrimental effects on the glymphatic system. His inability to get enough deep sleep is preventing the brain from effectively clearing amyloid-beta plaques, leading to their accumulation and subsequent cognitive decline. The chronic inflammation indicated by elevated CRP levels may further impair brain detox pathways, contributing to neuroinflammation and accelerated ageing.

Intervention:

The treatment plan for John would focus on improving sleep quality and restoring the brain's natural detoxification processes. Key steps include:

1. **Sleep Optimisation:** Implementing good sleep hygiene practices such as maintaining a regular sleep schedule, avoiding caffeine and alcohol before bed, and minimising exposure to screens and blue light in the evening.
2. **Melatonin Supplementation:** High-dose **melatonin** may be prescribed to regulate his circadian rhythm and enhance deep sleep.

3. **Cognitive Behavioural Therapy for Insomnia (CBT-I)**: John would benefit from behavioural strategies designed to reduce sleep anxiety and improve sleep quality over time.

4. **Anti-Inflammatory Support**: Addressing his elevated CRP levels with **anti-inflammatory supplements** like **omega-3 fatty acids** and **curcumin**, which have been shown to reduce neuroinflammation and support brain health.

5. **Mindfulness-Based Stress Reduction (MBSR)**: Incorporating mindfulness techniques to reduce overall stress, which may improve both his sleep quality and cognitive performance.

Outcome:

After implementing the treatment plan, John reports significant improvements in his sleep quality within six weeks. His total sleep time increases to an average of 7-8 hours per night, with more time spent in deep non-REM sleep. A follow-up neuroimaging scan shows a slight reduction in amyloid-beta accumulation, and his cognitive tests indicate improved memory retention and focus. He continues to practise mindfulness to manage his stress, and his inflammatory markers have reduced significantly.

Conclusion

The glymphatic system is the brain's essential waste clearance mechanism, functioning optimally during deep sleep. Disruptions to this system, caused by sleep deprivation or chronic inflammation, can lead to the buildup of toxic proteins like amyloid-beta, accelerating cognitive decline and increasing the risk of neurodegenerative diseases. Optimising sleep and supporting glymphatic function through lifestyle modifications, such as improving sleep hygiene and reducing stress, is a powerful way to maintain brain health and longevity.

By understanding the role of the glymphatic system and taking steps to ensure it functions properly, we can significantly reduce the risk of cognitive decline and enhance brain detoxification. Sleep is not just a time for rest but a critical period during which the brain cleanses itself of harmful waste—making it the foundation of cognitive resilience and mental clarity.

Toxic Proteins and Their Role in Neurodegeneration

Amyloid-Beta, Tau Proteins, and Alzheimer's Disease

Amyloid-beta and **tau proteins** are two of the most notorious culprits when it comes to the development of **Alzheimer's disease** and other neurodegenerative disorders. Understanding how these proteins contribute to brain toxicity and cognitive decline is essential in addressing brain health.

Amyloid-beta is a protein fragment produced as a byproduct of normal brain cell activity. In a healthy brain, amyloid beta is regularly cleared through the **glymphatic system**. However, when this process is compromised—whether due to poor sleep, ageing, or genetic factors—the clearance slows, leading to the accumulation of amyloid-beta in the spaces between neurons. These proteins clump together, forming **plaques** that disrupt neural communication and trigger inflammation. Over time, these plaques contribute to the progressive cognitive decline seen in Alzheimer's patients.

Similarly, **tau proteins**—which help maintain the structural integrity of neurons—can become dysfunctional. In Alzheimer's disease, tau proteins become **hyperphosphorylated**, meaning they have too many phosphate groups attached. This causes them to tangle inside neurons, leading to the formation of **neurofibrillary tangles**. These tangles interfere with the transport of nutrients and essential chemicals inside neurons, ultimately causing cell death. As more neurons die, brain regions responsible for memory, learning, and cognition begin to shrink, a hallmark of **brain atrophy** seen in advanced stages of Alzheimer's.

Both amyloid-beta and tau are naturally occurring proteins in the brain, but when their clearance and regulation break down, they become toxic and drive neurodegeneration. This makes **early intervention** crucial. Studies have shown that amyloid-beta accumulation can begin **decades** before cognitive symptoms appear, which is why optimising brain detox pathways through sleep, proper nutrition, and brain-boosting supplements is essential for prevention.

Recent therapies targeting amyloid-beta and tau, such as **monoclonal antibodies** designed to remove plaques or tau tangles, have shown promise. However, these treatments are often more effective in the early stages of Alzheimer's, when the toxic proteins are just beginning to accumulate. This highlights the importance of preventative strategies that support brain detox long before symptoms arise.

Environmental Toxins and Their Impact on the Brain

Beyond the brain's internal production of toxic proteins like amyloid-beta and tau, external **environmental toxins** also play a significant role in neurodegeneration. These toxins enter the body through various sources, including air pollution, contaminated water, pesticides in food, and chemicals in everyday products. Once inside the body, they can accumulate in the brain, disrupting normal function and contributing to cognitive decline.

One of the most well-documented environmental toxins affecting brain health is **mercury**, commonly found in certain fish, dental amalgams, and industrial pollution. Mercury can cross the **blood-brain barrier** and accumulate in the brain, where it damages neurons and impairs cellular processes. Studies have linked chronic mercury exposure to an increased risk of **Alzheimer's** and **Parkinson's disease**.

Another significant environmental toxin is **lead**, which widely used in paints and gasoline before its harmful effects were fully understood. Even today, traces of lead can be found in older homes, soil, and drinking water. Lead exposure during childhood is known to impair cognitive development, but it can also have long-term effects on adults, contributing to **neuroinflammation** and **cognitive decline**.

Air pollution is another growing concern for brain health. Studies show that individuals living in highly polluted areas are more likely to develop **neurodegenerative diseases** than those living in cleaner environments. Particulate matter in polluted air, including **heavy metals** and **organic compounds,** can penetrate the lungs and enter the bloodstream, eventually making its way to the brain. These pollutants trigger **oxidative stress,** neuroinflammation, and the buildup of toxic proteins, further accelerating the ageing process of the brain.

Pesticides and **herbicides** used in agriculture are also implicated in brain toxicity. **Organophosphates**, a class of pesticides, have been linked to neurodegenerative conditions, particularly **Parkinson's disease**. These chemicals disrupt the normal functioning of neurons, particularly those that produce **dopamine**, a neurotransmitter critical for movement and coordination.

Mitigating the impact of environmental toxins on brain health involves reducing exposure and supporting detoxification pathways. Dietary strategies such as consuming **antioxidant-rich foods** and **detoxifying herbs** like **cilantro**, **spirulina**, and **chlorella** can help remove heavy metals and other toxins from the body. Additionally, lifestyle changes—such as using air purifiers, drinking filtered water, and choosing organic produce—can limit toxin exposure and protect cognitive function.

Analogy: The Brain as a Factory—The Importance of Waste Disposal

Imagine the brain as a highly efficient factory, constantly working to produce thoughts, memories, decisions, and emotions. Just like any factory, the brain produces **waste** during its daily operations. This waste comes in the form of metabolic byproducts, such as **amyloid-beta** and **oxidised proteins**. In a healthy, well-functioning brain, these waste products are efficiently disposed of, ensuring the brain continues to run smoothly.

Now, think about what happens when a factory's waste disposal system breaks down. If garbage starts piling up on the factory floor, the workers (neurons) begin to slow down. They can't move as efficiently, and soon, the entire system grinds to a halt. In the same way, when the brain's **waste disposal system**—namely, the **glymphatic system** and other detox pathways—breaks down, harmful waste products accumulate, disrupting normal brain function.

Toxic proteins like **amyloid-beta** and **tau** are part of this accumulated waste. Normally, these proteins are cleared out by the glymphatic system during sleep, but when we don't get enough restorative sleep or when the detox system is overloaded with external toxins, these proteins build up, leading to **neuroinflammation** and the breakdown of neural connections. Over time, this results in cognitive decline and the onset of diseases like Alzheimer's.

In the analogy of the factory, the role of **sleep** is akin to the **night shift janitors** who come in and clean up the day's waste while the factory is shut down. Without them, the waste just keeps piling up. The same is true in the brain—deep sleep activates the glymphatic system, allowing it to clear away toxic proteins and maintain cognitive health.

Environmental toxins are like **industrial pollutants** that find their way into the factory and damage the machinery. When the brain is exposed to toxins like mercury, lead, or air pollution, the detox system is overwhelmed, and the "machinery" of the brain begins to break down, leading to oxidative stress and impaired neuron function. Over time, this accelerates the ageing process and increases the risk of neurodegenerative diseases.

To keep the brain's "factory" running efficiently, it's essential to maintain a **clean, healthy environment** both inside and outside the body. This means getting enough deep sleep to activate the glymphatic system, reducing exposure to environmental toxins, and supporting detoxification with proper nutrition and lifestyle choices.

Conclusion

The accumulation of toxic proteins like **amyloid-beta** and **tau**, along with the infiltration of **environmental toxins**, poses a significant threat to cognitive health. These harmful substances disrupt the brain's delicate balance, leading to neuroinflammation, oxidative stress, and ultimately neurodegeneration. By understanding the mechanisms behind protein toxicity and environmental damage, we can take proactive steps to support brain detoxification and protect cognitive function.

Addressing both **internal** and **external** sources of brain toxins is key to preventing neurodegenerative diseases and preserving long-term brain health. Optimising sleep, reducing environmental toxin exposure, and supporting detoxification pathways with targeted nutrition and supplementation are all essential strategies to maintain cognitive vitality and longevity.

Chronic Neuroinflammation: The Silent Threat to Brain Health

Microglial Cells and Brain Inflammation

At the heart of the brain's immune system are **microglial cells**, often referred to as the brain's **resident immune cells**. These cells play a dual role in maintaining brain health: they protect against infections and clear out debris and damaged cells through **phagocytosis**. In a healthy brain, microglial cells are constantly monitoring the environment, acting like sentinels to respond to any injury or infection. When functioning properly, microglial cells are crucial to brain detoxification, helping clear toxins and support neuron survival.

However, microglia can become overactive, leading to a state of **chronic neuroinflammation**. While short-term inflammation is a protective response to injury or infection, **long-term inflammation** within the brain becomes damaging. Overactive microglia release **pro-inflammatory cytokines** such as **tumour necrosis factor-alpha (TNF-α)** and **interleukin-6 (IL-6)**, which disrupt the communication between neurons, damage synapses, and impair brain detox pathways. As inflammation persists, microglia also release **reactive oxygen species (ROS)**, which cause oxidative stress and further damage neurons.

Chronic neuroinflammation is a silent threat because it often goes unnoticed until cognitive symptoms—such as memory loss, brain fog, and reduced mental clarity—become evident. Neuroinflammation is one of the early signs of **neurodegenerative diseases** like **Alzheimer's** and **Parkinson's**, as well as **depression** and other psychiatric disorders. Emerging research suggests that chronic neuroinflammation disrupts the **glymphatic system**, impairing the brain's ability to clear toxic proteins like amyloid-beta and tau, which in turn accelerates cognitive decline.

Ageing plays a major role in neuroinflammation. As we age, microglia become more sensitive to stimuli, resulting in an exaggerated inflammatory response even to minor injuries or stressors. This increased sensitivity, coupled with the slower ability of the brain to clear toxins, creates a vicious cycle of inflammation and cognitive deterioration.

Neuroinflammation is not limited to neurodegenerative diseases. Even in seemingly healthy individuals, chronic low-grade inflammation can impair cognitive performance. Conditions like **chronic stress**, **poor diet**, **sedentary lifestyle**, and **sleep deprivation** all contribute to the overactivation of microglia. Over time, this chronic neuroinflammatory state leads to neuronal damage and cognitive decline.

Case Study: Chronic Inflammation and Accelerated Aging

Patient Profile:

- **Name:** Sarah, age 62
- **Occupation:** Retired schoolteacher
- **Symptoms:** Memory problems, difficulty concentrating, frequent mental fatigue
- **Background:** Sarah led an active lifestyle during her working years but became more sedentary after retirement. She has a history of chronic stress due to family issues and often experiences poor sleep, getting only 4-5 hours of sleep per night. Over the past two years, she has noticed worsening memory and frequent mental fog. She feels fatigued after only short periods of mental activity and has difficulty remembering recent events.

Clinical Findings:

- Cognitive testing shows a decline in working memory and attention span.
- **Blood tests** reveal elevated levels of **C-reactive protein (CRP)** and **IL-6**, indicating systemic inflammation.
- **Neuroimaging** reveals signs of **brain atrophy**, particularly in the **hippocampus**, which is associated with memory formation.
- **Gut microbiome analysis** shows an imbalance of **gut bacteria**, with low levels of beneficial strains like **Bifidobacterium** and **Lactobacillus**, and an overgrowth of harmful bacteria.

Analysis:

Sarah's case highlights the cumulative impact of **chronic inflammation** on cognitive function. Her elevated inflammatory markers, such as CRP and IL-6, suggest that her immune system is in a persistent state of activation. This chronic inflammation has likely contributed to the atrophy in her hippocampus, a brain region crucial for memory. Additionally, her poor gut health, as indicated by the imbalance in her microbiome, may be exacerbating her neuroinflammatory state.

Her poor sleep patterns are another contributing factor. Sleep is critical for brain detoxification via the glymphatic system, and without sufficient deep sleep, Sarah's brain is unable to clear out the waste products and toxins that accumulate during the day. This combination of neuroinflammation, poor gut health, and inadequate sleep has accelerated the ageing process in her brain.

Intervention:

Sarah's treatment plan focuses on reducing systemic and neuroinflammation through a holistic approach:

1. **Anti-Inflammatory Diet**: Incorporating an **anti-inflammatory diet** rich in **omega-3 fatty acids** (found in fish and flaxseed), **antioxidants** (from colourful fruits and vegetables), and **polyphenols** (such as turmeric and green tea). This diet aims to reduce systemic inflammation and promote brain health.
2. **Probiotic Supplementation**: Restoring balance to her gut microbiome through the use of **probiotics** that contain strains like Bifidobacterium and Lactobacillus to reduce gut-driven inflammation.
3. **Sleep Optimisation**: Improving sleep hygiene to enhance deep sleep and activate the glymphatic system for brain detox. **Melatonin supplementation** may be introduced to help regulate her circadian rhythm.
4. **Mindfulness Meditation**: Incorporating **mindfulness practices** and **breathing exercises** to reduce chronic stress, a known contributor to neuroinflammation.
5. **Exercise**: Encouraging regular **aerobic exercise** and resistance training, which have been shown to reduce neuroinflammation and promote neurogenesis.

Outcome:

After three months of following the treatment plan, Sarah reports noticeable improvements in her cognitive function. She no longer experiences daily brain fog and has regained much of her mental clarity. Her sleep has improved significantly, with regular deep sleep allowing for more effective brain detoxification. Blood tests show a reduction in inflammatory markers (CRP and IL-6), and her gut microbiome has improved with higher levels of beneficial bacteria. Sarah continues to follow an anti-inflammatory diet and practice mindfulness to maintain these benefits.

Gut Health and Its Connection to Brain Detox

The link between the **gut** and the **brain**—often referred to as the **gut-brain axis**—is a key factor in understanding chronic neuroinflammation. The gut and the brain communicate bidirectionally through the **vagus nerve**, and the health of one often influences the health of the other. A growing body of research shows that **gut dysbiosis**—an imbalance in the gut microbiome—can trigger systemic inflammation, which in turn impacts the brain.

The **gut microbiome** consists of trillions of bacteria, fungi, and other microorganisms that reside in the digestive tract. These microorganisms play a crucial role in digestion, immune function, and even the production of **neurotransmitters** like serotonin and dopamine. However, when the balance of beneficial and harmful bacteria is disrupted, the gut becomes a source of inflammation. Harmful bacteria release **lipopolysaccharides (LPS)**, toxic molecules that enter the bloodstream and trigger an inflammatory response in the body and brain.

LPS has been shown to cross the **blood-brain barrier**, where it activates microglial cells and induces neuroinflammation. This cascade of inflammation not only disrupts normal brain function but also impairs the glymphatic system, making it harder for the brain to clear out toxic proteins like amyloid-beta. In this way, an unhealthy gut can directly contribute to cognitive decline and neurodegenerative diseases.

The state of the gut microbiome can also influence the production of **short-chain fatty acids (SCFAs)**, which have anti-inflammatory properties. Beneficial gut bacteria produce SCFAs like **butyrate**, which can reduce neuroinflammation and promote the health of brain cells. However, in cases of gut dysbiosis, the production of these SCFAs is reduced, leading to higher levels of inflammation both in the gut and the brain.

The connection between gut health and brain detox is further supported by the role of the **vagus nerve**, which acts as a communication highway between the gut and the central nervous system. The vagus nerve can be stimulated through practices like **deep breathing**, **cold exposure**, and **meditation**, all of which help reduce inflammation and promote the activation of the parasympathetic nervous system. When the vagus nerve is functioning optimally, it helps modulate the inflammatory response, reducing neuroinflammation and improving brain detox.

To optimise brain detox and reduce neuroinflammation, it is essential to prioritise gut health. This can be achieved through:

- **Probiotic supplementation** to restore the balance of the gut microbiome.
- **Prebiotic-rich foods** like garlic, onions, and asparagus, which feed beneficial gut bacteria.
- Avoiding **processed foods** and **sugar**, which promote gut dysbiosis.
- Consuming anti-inflammatory foods, particularly those rich in **fibre**, **polyphenols**, and **omega-3s**, which support gut and brain health.
- **Vagus nerve stimulation** techniques to enhance the gut-brain connection and reduce systemic inflammation.

Conclusion

Chronic neuroinflammation is a silent yet powerful force driving cognitive decline and neurodegenerative diseases. The overactivation of **microglial cells**, triggered by factors such as ageing, stress, and poor gut health, can disrupt brain detox pathways, leading to the accumulation of toxic proteins and the deterioration of cognitive function. Addressing neuroinflammation through a combination of **anti-inflammatory diets**, **gut health optimisation**, and **lifestyle interventions** is essential for promoting brain health and longevity.

The **gut-brain axis** plays a crucial role in regulating inflammation, and by supporting a healthy gut microbiome, we can reduce systemic inflammation and enhance the brain's ability to detoxify and heal. The interplay between the gut and brain highlights the importance of a holistic approach to brain health—one that considers both the body and the mind.

Summary: The Glymphatic System: The Brain's Cleansing Mechanism

(a) Glymphatic Syste

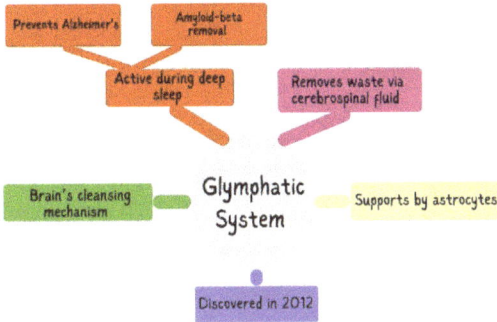

(b) Role of Sleep in Detox

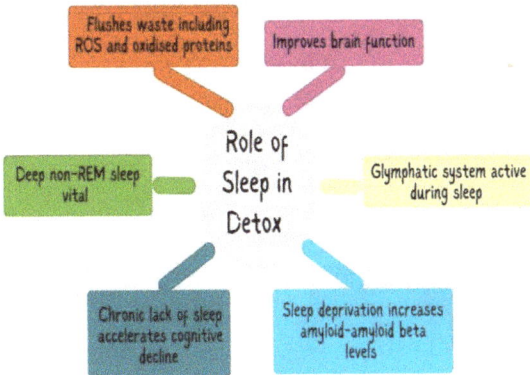

(c) Toxic Proteins and Neuro-Degeneration

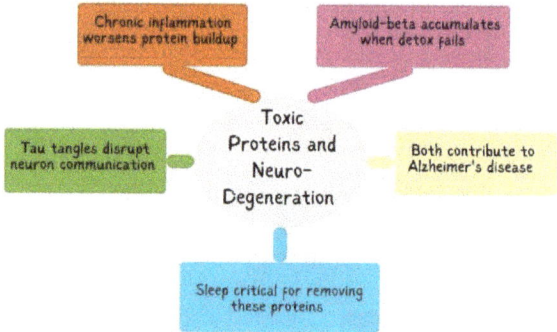

- Chronic inflammation worsens protein buildup
- Amyloid-beta accumulates when detox fails
- Tau tangles disrupt neuron communication
- Toxic Proteins and Neuro-Degeneration
- Both contribute to Alzheimer's disease
- Sleep critical for removing these proteins

(d) Environmental Toxins and Brain Health

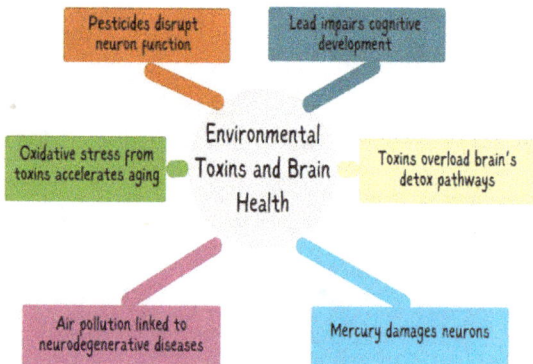

- Pesticides disrupt neuron function
- Lead impairs cognitive development
- Oxidative stress from toxins accelerates aging
- Environmental Toxins and Brain Health
- Toxins overload brain's detox pathways
- Air pollution linked to neurodegenerative diseases
- Mercury damages neurons

Chapter Two: NAD+, Procaine, and CoQ10: Modern Molecules for Neuroprotection

The Role of NAD+ in Cellular Energy and Detox

NAD+ (Nicotinamide Adenine Dinucleotide) is a critical molecule that serves as a coenzyme in numerous metabolic processes, playing a vital role in energy production and cellular repair. NAD+ is often described as the "fuel" for cellular energy, as it is directly involved in **mitochondrial function**, where energy in the form of **ATP (adenosine triphosphate)** is produced. In addition to its energy-regulating functions, NAD+ is central to cellular detoxification and repair mechanisms, including the **activation of sirtuins**, a family of proteins that regulate cellular health and longevity.

One of the most critical roles NAD+ plays in brain health is its ability to support **DNA repair** and prevent **oxidative damage**. Every day, cells are exposed to oxidative stress caused by free radicals, which can damage DNA and other cellular structures. NAD+ works with proteins such as **PARPs (Poly ADP-ribose polymerases)** to repair DNA and reduce cellular dysfunction. Without sufficient NAD+ levels, this repair process slows, leading to **cellular senescence** (ageing) and impaired brain function.

In the context of brain detoxification, NAD+ promotes **autophagy**, the process by which cells degrade and recycle their own damaged or unnecessary components, including dysfunctional proteins and organelles. Autophagy is critical in neuroprotection, as it helps clear out toxic proteins like **amyloid-beta** and **tau**, which are associated with **Alzheimer's disease** and other neurodegenerative conditions. When NAD+ levels are optimised, brain cells (neurons) become more efficient at removing waste, reducing the likelihood of neurodegeneration.

However, NAD+ levels naturally decline with age. By the time individuals reach their 40s and 50s, NAD+ levels may be reduced by nearly 50%. This decline in NAD+ contributes to mitochondrial dysfunction, impaired cellular detox, and an increased risk of cognitive decline. Fortunately, modern therapies aimed at **restoring NAD+ levels** through supplementation or **NAD+ infusions** have shown promise in supporting brain health and reversing aspects of age-related cognitive impairment.

Neuroscience Insight: NAD+ and Mitochondrial Health

The mitochondria, often referred to as the **powerhouses of the cell**, are responsible for generating the energy needed for all cellular functions. The brain, being one of the most metabolically active organs, depends heavily on mitochondria for optimal function. NAD+ is essential for the proper functioning of mitochondria, as it fuels the reactions that generate ATP.

In recent years, research has demonstrated that **mitochondrial dysfunction** is a key factor in the progression of neurodegenerative diseases like Alzheimer's, Parkinson's, and ALS. When mitochondria are not functioning optimally, they produce less energy and generate more **reactive oxygen species (ROS)**, which leads to oxidative damage and inflammation within the brain. This creates a feedback loop of damage that accelerates neuronal death and cognitive decline.

NAD+ helps mitigate this damage by supporting the function of **sirtuins**, a group of enzymes that protect mitochondria from stress and promote their repair. **SIRT1**, a well-known member of this enzyme family, is activated by NAD+ and has been shown to extend lifespan in animal models by enhancing mitochondrial function and reducing oxidative stress. Additionally, NAD+ promotes the process of **mitophagy**, a specific form of autophagy that removes damaged mitochondria, preventing them from releasing harmful byproducts.

By boosting NAD+ levels, either through supplementation or intravenous infusions, we can enhance mitochondrial function, improve energy production, and protect neurons from oxidative damage. Clinical studies have shown that NAD+ restoration can lead to improvements in cognitive performance, energy levels, and overall brain health, making it a key component in the fight against neurodegeneration.

Case History: NAD+ Infusions and Cognitive Decline

Patient Profile:

- **Name**: Michael, age 64
- **Occupation**: Retired engineer
- **Symptoms**: Memory loss, reduced mental clarity, fatigue
- **Background**: Michael had been noticing gradual cognitive decline for several years, with increasing difficulty remembering names, focusing on complex tasks, and experiencing mental fatigue after short periods of concentration. He has no family history of dementia but has a history of chronic stress and poor sleep. His lifestyle has become more sedentary in recent years.

Clinical Findings:

- **Cognitive assessments** showed mild cognitive impairment, with declines in **short-term memory** and **executive function**.
- **Blood tests** revealed low NAD+ levels and elevated **oxidative stress markers**.
- **Neuroimaging** showed minor atrophy in the **hippocampus**, the area of the brain responsible for memory formation.

Intervention:

Given Michael's symptoms and test results, his physician recommended a course of **NAD+ intravenous infusions** to restore his mitochondrial function and improve cellular detoxification. The treatment plan involved:

1. **NAD+ Infusions**: Michael received bi-weekly intravenous infusions of NAD+ over six weeks. The goal was to replenish his NAD+ levels, support mitochondrial health, and enhance brain detox processes like autophagy.
2. **Lifestyle Modifications**: He was encouraged to adopt a **Mediterranean diet**, rich in **omega-3 fatty acids** and antioxidants, to further support brain health and reduce inflammation.
3. **Exercise Program**: A moderate exercise program focusing on **aerobic exercise** and resistance training was introduced to stimulate mitochondrial activity and reduce cognitive fatigue.

Outcome:

After completing the six-week NAD+ infusion therapy, Michael reported significant improvements in his mental clarity, memory, and overall energy levels. His cognitive testing showed a reversal of some of his impairments, and his oxidative stress markers were reduced. Neuroimaging conducted three months later showed no further hippocampal atrophy, and his physician noted a marked improvement in mitochondrial function and detox efficiency. Michael continues to receive NAD+ infusions quarterly to maintain these benefits.

Procaine as a Regenerative Biohack

Procaine, an anaesthetic developed in the early 20th century, has more recently gained attention for its **regenerative** properties, particularly in Europe, where it has been used in **bioregulatory medicine**. Procaine is not only used for its numbing effects but also for its ability to **regenerate cells**, improve **blood circulation**, and support **neurological health.**

When administered in small doses, procaine has been found to stabilise cell membranes, reduce oxidative stress, and improve cellular communication. It enhances **DNA repair** processes, much like NAD+, by reducing the formation of harmful free radicals. Procaine also supports **nerve regeneration**, making it a useful treatment for neurodegenerative conditions and age-related cognitive decline.

One of the mechanisms by which procaine exerts its neuroprotective effects is by improving the function of the **mitochondria** and enhancing cellular detoxification pathways. Like NAD+, procaine helps promote autophagy, ensuring that damaged proteins and organelles are efficiently removed from the brain, reducing the risk of neurodegenerative disease.

Procaine's regenerative effects have been harnessed in treatments like **neural therapy**, where it is injected into specific points of the body to restore balance to the autonomic nervous system, reduce chronic pain, and improve brain function. Although research on procaine's role in neuroprotection is still emerging, early results are promising, especially when combined with other regenerative biohacks like **NAD+** and **CoQ10.**

CoQ10's Role in Enhancing Mitochondrial Function

CoQ10 (Coenzyme Q10) is a naturally occurring antioxidant that plays a vital role in the production of energy within cells, particularly in the mitochondria. CoQ10 acts as an **electron carrier** in the mitochondrial respiratory chain, facilitating the production of ATP, the energy currency of the cell. It is also one of the body's most powerful **antioxidants**, neutralising free radicals and reducing oxidative stress.

In the brain, CoQ10 is crucial for maintaining healthy mitochondrial function, which is essential for cognitive performance and neuroprotection. As we age, the body's natural levels of CoQ10 decline, leading to reduced energy production, mitochondrial dysfunction, and increased oxidative damage. This decline in CoQ10 has been linked to a higher risk of **Alzheimer's disease**, **Parkinson's disease**, and other age-related neurodegenerative conditions.

Supplementing with CoQ10 can help reverse these age-related declines by enhancing mitochondrial efficiency, reducing oxidative damage, and improving brain detoxification. CoQ10 also helps stabilise cell membranes, protecting neurons from damage caused by oxidative stress and inflammation. In clinical trials, CoQ10 supplementation has been shown to slow the progression of neurodegenerative diseases and improve cognitive function in ageing individuals.

Analogy: CoQ10 is the Engine Oil of the Brain

Think of CoQ10 as the **engine oil** for the brain's mitochondria. Just like a car engine needs oil to run smoothly and prevent wear and tear, the brain's mitochondria need CoQ10 to function efficiently and produce energy without generating excessive free radicals. When the engine oil is low, the engine overheats wears out faster and eventually breaks down. Similarly, when CoQ10 levels are low, the brain's mitochondria produce less energy and generate more oxidative damage, accelerating the ageing process and cognitive decline.

By supplementing with CoQ10, we're essentially **topping up the brain's oil**, ensuring that the mitochondria can continue to produce energy efficiently while reducing oxidative stress. This protects neurons from damage and supports the detoxification processes that are vital for maintaining cognitive health as we age.

Conclusion

NAD+, procaine, and CoQ10 represent a powerful trio of modern molecules that can significantly enhance brain health and neuroprotection. NAD+ is critical for mitochondrial function and cellular detox, while procaine offers regenerative benefits by improving cell communication and reducing oxidative stress. CoQ10, as a potent antioxidant and mitochondrial enhancer, acts like the brain's engine oil, ensuring smooth and efficient energy production.

Together, these molecules offer a multi-faceted approach to slowing cognitive decline, supporting brain detoxification, and enhancing mitochondrial function—key strategies for maintaining cognitive longevity and protecting against neurodegenerative diseases.

Jim Kwik's Cognitive Biohacks: The Power of Monotasking

Why Multitasking Is Inefficient

In today's fast-paced digital world, **multitasking** has become the norm. People pride themselves on juggling multiple tasks at once—checking emails while attending meetings, browsing social media while working, and constantly switching between projects. While multitasking may seem like an efficient way to accomplish more, neuroscience tells a different story.

Multitasking is not only inefficient, but it also significantly **impairs cognitive performance**. Research has shown that the human brain is not wired to handle multiple tasks simultaneously. When we attempt to multitask, what we're doing is **task-switching**, which involves rapidly shifting attention between tasks rather than performing them simultaneously. This switching process requires cognitive energy and disrupts focus, leading to **mental fatigue** and a decline in the quality of work.

The **prefrontal cortex**, the brain's executive centre responsible for decision-making, focus, and higher-order thinking, becomes overwhelmed when forced to manage several tasks at once. Each time we switch tasks, the brain requires time to reorient and refocus, which reduces efficiency. Studies have shown that it can take up to **23 minutes** to fully refocus after switching tasks, meaning valuable time is lost in the process. Over time, multitasking leads to **cognitive overload**, increased stress, and a greater likelihood of making mistakes.

Moreover, multitasking harms **memory** and **learning**. When the brain is constantly shifting focus, it doesn't have time to consolidate information or transfer knowledge from **short-term memory** to **long-term memory**. This is why people often forget details or struggle to retain new information when they're multitasking.

In contrast, **monotasking**—the practice of focusing on one task at a time—allows the brain to work at its highest level of efficiency. By dedicating full attention to a single task, cognitive resources are optimised, and deeper, more meaningful work is accomplished. Monotasking also reduces **mental clutter**, enabling clearer thinking, better decision-making, and improved productivity.

Techniques to Improve Focus and Mental Clarity

Shifting from a multitasking mindset to a **monotasking** approach requires a change in habits and mindset, but the benefits to cognitive health and productivity are well worth it. Below are some of Jim Kwik's most effective **cognitive biohacks** for improving focus, mental clarity, and productivity through monotasking.

1. Time Blocking:
   One of the most effective monotasking techniques is **time blocking**—dedicating specific periods to focus on a single task without distractions. During these blocks, turn off notifications, close unrelated tabs, and focus solely on the task at hand. Jim Kwik recommends the **Pomodoro Technique**, which involves working in 25-minute intervals followed by a short break. This method takes advantage of the brain's natural focus rhythms, helping to sustain attention and reduce burnout.

2. Eliminate Digital Distractions:
   Digital distractions are a major culprit of multitasking. To successfully monotask, it's important to **limit screen time** and digital interruptions. Start by turning off non-essential notifications on your phone and computer, and designate specific times to check emails and social media. This allows your brain to focus on work without the constant temptation of switching to another task. Jim Kwik also suggests using **focus-enhancing apps** that block distractions, such as Freedom or Cold Turkey, to help maintain concentration.

3. Set Clear Goals:
   Without clear goals, the brain tends to wander, leading to unproductive multitasking. Setting **specific, achievable goals** for each work session helps the brain stay focused and prevents mental drift. Break down large tasks into smaller, manageable parts, and tackle them one at a time. This provides a sense of accomplishment and helps maintain momentum, which is key to staying in a focused state.

4. Mindful Transitions:
   Task-switching is unavoidable in some cases, but the way we transition between tasks can make a significant difference in cognitive performance. Jim Kwik advises practising **mindful transitions**—taking a moment to breathe and reset between tasks rather than jumping from one activity to another. This helps clear mental clutter and allows the brain to refocus on the next task with renewed energy.

5. Brain Breaks:
   The brain cannot focus for extended periods without breaks. Research shows that the brain's ability to concentrate diminishes after about 45-60 minutes of intense focus. Jim Kwik recommends incorporating **brain breaks**—short periods of relaxation or movement—between work sessions to recharge. These breaks allow the brain to reset, improve memory retention, and increase creativity.

6. Visualisation and Mental Rehearsal:
    Jim Kwik is a strong advocate of **visualisation techniques** to enhance focus and productivity. Before starting a task, take a moment to visualise yourself completing it successfully. Mentally rehearsing the process primes the brain for success and helps you stay engaged and motivated. This cognitive biohack is especially useful for tasks that require creative thinking or problem-solving.

7. Focus-Enhancing Nutrition:
    Diet plays a significant role in cognitive performance. Jim Kwik emphasises the importance of **brain-boosting foods** such as **omega-3 fatty acids,** found in fish, flaxseeds, and walnuts, which support brain health and improve focus. Additionally, **antioxidant-rich foods** like berries and dark chocolate protect the brain from oxidative stress and enhance mental clarity. Kwik also suggests staying hydrated and avoiding processed foods and sugars, which can lead to brain fog and reduced concentration.

8. Sleep Optimisation:
    A rested brain is a focused brain. Jim Kwik emphasises the importance of getting **quality sleep** to improve focus, memory, and mental clarity. During sleep, the brain consolidates memories and clears out toxins through the **glymphatic system,** preparing the mind for optimal performance the next day. By prioritising 7-9 hours of quality sleep each night, you set the stage for effective monotasking the following day.

By adopting these monotasking techniques, you can train your brain to focus more effectively, reduce mental fatigue, and improve overall cognitive performance.

Case Study: Enhancing Productivity Through Monotasking

Patient Profile:

- **Name**: Lisa, age 35
- **Occupation**: Marketing manager at a digital advertising agency
- **Symptoms**: Frequent distractions, difficulty focusing, decreased productivity, mental fatigue
- **Background**: Lisa has always been a high achiever, but recently she has struggled to keep up with the demands of her job. Between managing multiple projects, attending meetings, and constantly checking her phone and emails, she feels overwhelmed and mentally exhausted by the end of the day. She's noticed that her productivity has dropped, and she often forgets important details or makes mistakes in her work. Lisa reports spending 10-12 hours a day in front of a screen and feels that her work quality has diminished.

Clinical Findings:

- **Cognitive tests** revealed impairments in **working memory** and **sustained attention**, both of which are essential for multitasking effectively.
- A survey of Lisa's daily habits shows that she switches tasks more than 50 times per day and spends less than 15 minutes on any one project before being interrupted by emails, messages, or meetings.
- Her **stress levels** are elevated, and she reports feeling mentally drained by mid-afternoon, despite spending long hours on the job.

Intervention:

Lisa's situation is a classic case of **cognitive overload** caused by chronic multitasking. Her brain is constantly being forced to switch between tasks, leading to reduced productivity, increased mental fatigue, and errors in her work. To improve her focus and productivity, Lisa was introduced to Jim Kwik's **monotasking biohacks**.

Time Blocking: Lisa began using the **Pomodoro Technique**, working in 25-minute intervals with 5-minute breaks in between. During these work blocks, she focused on one project at a time, turning off her phone and email notifications to minimise distractions.

1.

   Digital Detox: Lisa designated specific times during the day to check her emails and messages, rather than responding to them as they arrived. This helped her maintain focus during her work blocks without constant interruptions.

2. **Mindful Transitions**: Lisa practised deep breathing exercises for 2-3 minutes between tasks to reset her mind and reduce stress. This allowed her to approach each new task with fresh energy and focus.

   Brain Breaks: To combat mental fatigue, Lisa incorporated short walks or stretching exercises during her breaks. This helped improve her mental clarity and prevented burnout by the end of the day.

3. **Goal Setting**: Each morning, Lisa set clear goals for the day, outlining the top 3 tasks she wanted to complete by the end of the day. This gave her a sense of direction and helped her avoid task-switching.

Outcome:

After implementing these monotasking techniques for one month, Lisa noticed significant improvements in her focus, productivity, and mental clarity. She was able to complete projects more efficiently and made fewer mistakes in her work. Her workday was shortened from 10-12 hours to a more manageable 8 hours, as she no longer wasted time switching between tasks. Additionally, Lisa reported feeling less mentally exhausted by the end of the day and was able to enjoy more quality time outside of work.

Conclusion

Monotasking is a powerful cognitive biohack that enhances mental clarity, focus, and productivity. By focusing on one task at a time, eliminating distractions, and adopting strategies like time blocking and mindful transitions, individuals can overcome the inefficiencies of multitasking and achieve deeper, more meaningful work. As Lisa's case demonstrates, implementing these monotasking techniques can lead to improved productivity, reduced mental fatigue, and a more balanced work-life dynamic.

Incorporating these biohacks into your daily routine will allow you to **optimise brain function**, reduce stress, and tap into your full cognitive potential. Monotasking is not just about getting more done—it's about doing better work with less mental strain.

Nootropics: Enhancing Brain Detox with Smart Supplements

Bacopa Monnieri, Lion's Mane, Omega-3, Rhodiola

Nootropics, often referred to as "smart supplements," are natural or synthetic compounds that enhance brain function. These substances have gained immense popularity due to their ability to boost memory, focus, learning capacity, and mental clarity while supporting brain detoxification. A growing body of scientific research shows that certain nootropics can protect neurons, reduce oxidative stress, and promote **neuroplasticity**, the brain's ability to reorganise itself by forming new neural connections. This section focuses on four powerful nootropics—**Bacopa Monnieri, Lion's Mane, Omega-3 fatty acids**, and **Rhodiola**—and their role in improving brain health and cognitive function.

Bacopa Monnieri: The Memory Booster

Bacopa Monnieri is an ancient herb used in **Ayurvedic medicine** for centuries as a brain tonic. Modern research supports its traditional use, showing that Bacopa enhances memory, cognitive function, and brain detoxification. The active compounds in Bacopa, known as **bacosides**, have been found to improve **synaptic communication**, enhance memory retention, and reduce the build-up of toxic proteins in the brain, such as **amyloid-beta**, which contributes to **Alzheimer's disease**.

Bacopa works by increasing the production of **acetylcholine**, a neurotransmitter associated with learning and memory. Additionally, it promotes the repair of damaged neurons by enhancing synaptic plasticity, making it an effective supplement for both brain detox and cognitive enhancement. Studies have shown that Bacopa can reduce **cognitive decline** in elderly individuals, while also improving **working memory** and **executive function** in younger populations.

Bacopa Monnieri also acts as an **antioxidant**, reducing oxidative stress in the brain, which is crucial for preventing **neuroinflammation**. Its ability to neutralise free radicals and support the body's detoxification pathways makes it a powerful nootropic for long-term brain health.

Lion's Mane: The Neuroplasticity Enhancer

Lion's Mane Mushroom (Hericium erinaceus) has gained a reputation as one of the most potent nootropics for enhancing **neuroplasticity**—the brain's ability to grow and adapt throughout life. Lion's Mane is rich in compounds called **hericenones** and **erinacines**, which stimulate the production of **nerve growth factor (NGF)**, a protein essential for the growth, maintenance, and survival of neurons.

Neuroplasticity is essential for brain detox because it allows the brain to form new connections, repair damaged neurons, and clear out toxic proteins. Lion's Mane's ability to enhance NGF production makes it particularly effective in supporting **cognitive function**, memory, and learning, while also reducing the risk of **neurodegenerative diseases** like **Alzheimer's** and **Parkinson's disease**.

Lion's Mane has also been shown to reduce **symptoms of anxiety and depression**, both of which are linked to brain inflammation and oxidative stress. By reducing inflammation and supporting brain detox pathways, Lion's Mane helps protect the brain from long-term damage while promoting mental clarity and focus.

In animal studies, Lion's Mane has been found to reduce **amyloid-beta plaques** in the brain, improve cognitive function, and reverse memory deficits. These findings suggest that Lion's Mane could play a role in both the prevention and treatment of neurodegenerative conditions.

Omega-3 Fatty Acids: The Brain's Building Blocks

Omega-3 fatty acids, particularly **DHA (docosahexaenoic acid)** and **EPA (eicosapentaenoic acid)**, are essential for brain health. DHA makes up a significant portion of the brain's grey matter and is crucial for maintaining the structure and function of brain cells. Omega-3s are also known for their potent anti-inflammatory effects, which help reduce **neuroinflammation**—a key driver of cognitive decline and neurodegenerative diseases.

Omega-3 fatty acids play a critical role in **brain detoxification** by supporting the integrity of the **blood-brain barrier** (BBB), a protective layer that prevents toxins and harmful substances from entering the brain. When the BBB is compromised, toxins can infiltrate the brain, leading to inflammation and the accumulation of harmful proteins like **amyloid-beta**. Omega-3s help maintain the health of the BBB, ensuring that the brain remains protected from environmental toxins.

In addition to protecting the BBB, Omega-3s enhance **mitochondrial function**, supporting the brain's energy production and reducing oxidative stress. Studies have shown that individuals with higher levels of DHA and EPA have better cognitive function, memory retention, and a lower risk of developing **Alzheimer's disease**.

Omega-3 supplementation has also been linked to improved **mood and mental clarity**, making it an essential component of any brain-boosting regimen. For optimal brain health, Omega-3s can be obtained through dietary sources such as **fatty fish**, **flaxseeds**, **chia seeds**, or high-quality fish oil supplements.

Rhodiola: The Adaptogen for Cognitive Resilience

Rhodiola Rosea is a powerful **adaptogen**—a natural substance that helps the body adapt to stress and maintain balance. Rhodiola has long been used in traditional medicine to enhance mental and physical endurance, reduce fatigue, and improve cognitive function. Its cognitive benefits are largely due to its ability to modulate the release of **stress hormones** like **cortisol** while also promoting **neurotransmitter balance**.

Chronic stress is one of the biggest contributors to neuroinflammation and cognitive decline. When the body is under constant stress, cortisol levels rise, which can impair memory, reduce focus, and increase the accumulation of toxic proteins in the brain. Rhodiola helps buffer the brain against these harmful effects by reducing cortisol levels and enhancing **dopamine** and **serotonin** activity, two neurotransmitters essential for mood regulation and mental clarity.

Rhodiola's antioxidant properties further support brain detox by reducing oxidative damage and promoting cellular repair. It has been shown to improve **working memory**, enhance **mental clarity**, and boost **cognitive resilience** in the face of stress. For individuals experiencing burnout, fatigue, or cognitive fog, Rhodiola offers a natural way to restore mental vitality and protect the brain from stress-induced damage.

Case Study: Nootropics and Mental Clarity

Patient Profile:

- **Name**: Emily, age 45
- **Occupation**: Accountant
- **Symptoms**: Brain fog, difficulty concentrating, frequent mental fatigue
- **Background**: Emily has been working in a demanding accounting role for over 15 years. Recently, she has noticed a significant decline in her ability to focus on complex tasks and maintain mental clarity throughout the day. She experiences brain fog, particularly in the afternoon, and often struggles to recall details during meetings. Emily reports feeling mentally drained by the end of the workday, despite getting 7-8 hours of sleep each night.

Clinical Findings:

- **Cognitive testing** revealed mild deficits in **executive function** and **working memory**, two areas essential for performing the detailed work required in her profession.
- **Nutrient testing** showed low levels of **omega-3 fatty acids** and moderate **oxidative stress**, likely contributing to her cognitive symptoms.
- Emily's **stress levels** were elevated, indicating that her body was in a state of chronic low-level stress, contributing to her brain fog and mental fatigue.

Intervention:

Emily's treatment plan focused on introducing **nootropics** that would enhance her cognitive function, support brain detox, and reduce mental fatigue. The following nootropics were recommended:

1. **Omega-3 Supplementation**: Emily began taking a daily **omega-3 supplement** containing high levels of **DHA** and **EPA** to support brain structure, reduce oxidative stress, and improve mental clarity.

2. **Bacopa Monnieri**: A **Bacopa Monnieri** extract was introduced to enhance her memory retention and promote synaptic plasticity. The antioxidant properties of Bacopa were also expected to reduce the buildup of oxidative waste in her brain.

3. **Lion's Mane**: Emily started taking a daily dose of **Lion's Mane** to stimulate nerve growth factor (NGF) production, support neuroplasticity, and improve her overall cognitive function.

4. **Rhodiola Rosea**: To combat stress and mental fatigue, **Rhodiola** was included in her regimen. This adaptogen would help regulate her cortisol levels, increase her mental resilience, and restore cognitive vitality.

Outcome:

After three months of following her nootropic regimen, Emily reported significant improvements in her mental clarity and focus. Her brain fog had diminished, and she was able to perform complex accounting tasks with greater ease and precision. Emily's energy levels improved, allowing her to remain mentally sharp throughout the workday. Cognitive testing showed enhanced executive function and working memory, and her stress levels had decreased, contributing to her overall sense of well-being.

Conclusion

Nootropics such as **Bacopa Monnieri**, **Lion's Mane**, **Omega-3 fatty acids**, and **Rhodiola** offer powerful support for brain detoxification, cognitive enhancement, and mental clarity. These smart supplements not only boost cognitive performance but also protect the brain from the harmful effects of oxidative stress, neuroinflammation, and the accumulation of toxic proteins.

By integrating nootropics into a daily regimen, individuals can improve focus, memory, and mental resilience, while also enhancing the brain's natural detox pathways. Whether you are looking to prevent cognitive decline, combat brain fog, or simply optimise your mental performance, nootropics provide a safe and effective solution for long-term brain health.

High-Dose Melatonin: A Sleep and Brain Detox Superpower

Sleep and Its Role in Brain Detox

Sleep is one of the most powerful tools for maintaining brain health and promoting detoxification. During deep sleep, the brain undergoes a critical process of **cleansing**, facilitated by the **glymphatic system**, which removes waste products, including toxic proteins like **amyloid-beta** and **tau**, that accumulate throughout the day. These proteins, if not efficiently cleared, can form plaques and tangles, contributing to neurodegenerative diseases like **Alzheimer's** and **Parkinson's disease**.

The glymphatic system is most active during **non-REM sleep**, particularly in the **deep stages of sleep**. During this time, the brain's cells shrink, creating space for **cerebrospinal fluid (CSF)** to flow more freely through the brain tissue, effectively flushing out harmful toxins and metabolic waste. This process plays a critical role in preventing cognitive decline and maintaining overall brain health.

However, many people do not get enough deep sleep due to stress, poor sleep habits, or underlying health conditions. Over time, chronic sleep deprivation impairs the glymphatic system's ability to clear toxins, leading to the buildup of **neurotoxins** and an increased risk of cognitive decline. This is where **melatonin**, particularly in high doses, can play a transformative role in brain detoxification and neuroprotection.

Melatonin, a hormone produced by the **pineal gland,** regulates the sleep-wake cycle and is often referred to as the "sleep hormone." Its production naturally increases in response to darkness, signalling the body to prepare for sleep. However, in modern society, exposure to artificial light, especially from screens, can disrupt melatonin production, resulting in poor sleep quality.

In addition to regulating sleep, melatonin is a powerful **antioxidant** that protects the brain from oxidative stress and inflammation. It crosses the **blood-brain barrier,** directly neutralising free radicals and reducing oxidative damage to neurons. This dual role as both a sleep regulator and antioxidant makes melatonin particularly valuable for brain detox.

Recent research has shown that **high-dose melatonin** can significantly enhance deep sleep and glymphatic activity, thereby improving the brain's ability to clear toxins. High-dose melatonin not only enhances the duration of deep sleep but also amplifies the glymphatic system's efficiency, allowing for a more thorough clearance of toxic proteins that contribute to cognitive decline.

Melatonin's neuroprotective properties extend beyond its role in sleep regulation. Studies have found that melatonin can **reduce amyloid-beta accumulation** in the brain, slow down the progression of **Alzheimer's disease,** and improve cognitive function in individuals with **mild cognitive impairment (MCI).** These effects make melatonin a promising supplement for those looking to enhance brain detoxification and protect against neurodegeneration.

Case Study: Melatonin and Dementia Prevention

Patient Profile:

- **Name:** Margaret, age 72
- **Occupation:** Retired teacher
- **Symptoms:** Memory lapses, difficulty sleeping, daytime fatigue, mild cognitive impairment

- **Background**: Margaret began experiencing sleep disturbances in her late 60s, initially chalking it up to stress and ageing. Over the past few years, however, she noticed an increase in memory problems, including difficulty recalling recent conversations and struggling to remember appointments. These cognitive issues were accompanied by frequent daytime fatigue, which left her feeling drained and unable to fully enjoy her retirement. Margaret had a family history of **Alzheimer's disease**, which raised concerns about her long-term brain health.

Clinical Findings:

- Cognitive tests showed early signs of mild cognitive impairment (MCI), particularly in short-term memory and executive function.
- A **polysomnography study** revealed fragmented sleep patterns with reduced time spent in **deep non-REM sleep**, which is critical for brain detoxification.
- Blood tests indicated low levels of **melatonin** production, particularly during the night, likely contributing to her poor sleep quality.
- **Neuroimaging** revealed the early buildup of **amyloid-beta plaques** in the brain, a hallmark of Alzheimer's disease.

Analysis:

Margaret's case highlighted the connection between poor sleep, reduced melatonin production, and the early signs of cognitive decline. Her inability to achieve deep, restorative sleep was impairing the glymphatic system's ability to clear amyloid-beta and other toxic proteins from her brain. As a result, these toxins were beginning to accumulate, leading to memory issues and increasing her risk of Alzheimer's disease. Given her family history of dementia, early intervention was critical.

Intervention:

Margaret's treatment plan focused on restoring her sleep quality and enhancing her brain's detoxification processes using **high-dose melatonin supplementation**. The key components of her treatment plan included:

1. **High-Dose Melatonin Supplementation**: Margaret was prescribed **20 mg of melatonin** each night, taken 30 minutes before bedtime. This higher-than-average dose was aimed at boosting her body's natural melatonin levels, promoting deeper sleep, and enhancing the glymphatic system's function.

2. **Sleep Hygiene Optimisation**: In addition to melatonin supplementation, Margaret adopted several **sleep hygiene practices** to improve her sleep environment. These included maintaining a consistent sleep schedule, avoiding blue light from screens at least two hours before bed, and creating a dark, cool, and quiet sleep environment.

3. **Anti-Inflammatory Diet**: Margaret was encouraged to follow an **anti-inflammatory diet**, rich in **omega-3 fatty acids**, **antioxidants**, and **polyphenols** to reduce neuroinflammation and support brain health. Foods like **salmon, blueberries**, and **turmeric** were emphasised for their neuroprotective properties.

4. **Mindfulness and Stress Reduction**: To address underlying stress and anxiety, Margaret began practising **mindfulness meditation** and **deep breathing exercises**. These techniques helped reduce her overall stress levels, which contributed to better sleep quality and cognitive resilience.

5. **Cognitive Exercises**: To stimulate her brain and improve memory, Margaret was also encouraged to engage in **cognitive exercises**, such as puzzles, memory games, and reading, to strengthen neural connections and improve brain plasticity.

Outcome:

After three months of high-dose melatonin supplementation and implementing sleep hygiene practices, Margaret reported significant improvements in her sleep quality. She was able to fall asleep more easily and experienced fewer nighttime awakenings. Importantly, her time spent in deep sleep, as measured by a follow-up sleep study, had increased by 40%, allowing for more effective brain detoxification.

In addition to better sleep, Margaret noticed improvements in her cognitive function. Her memory lapses became less frequent, and she felt more mentally alert during the day. Follow-up cognitive testing showed a modest improvement in her executive function and short-term memory, suggesting that her cognitive decline had stabilised.

Most notably, a follow-up neuroimaging scan revealed a reduction in amyloid-beta accumulation, indicating that the enhanced glymphatic clearance during sleep was helping to slow the progression of Alzheimer's disease. While Margaret remained vigilant about her brain health, the improvements in her sleep and cognition gave her a sense of control over her long-term mental well-being.

Conclusion

High-dose melatonin is a powerful tool for enhancing brain detox and preventing cognitive decline. By promoting deeper, more restorative sleep, melatonin optimises the glymphatic system's ability to clear toxic proteins from the brain, protecting against neurodegenerative diseases like Alzheimer's. In addition to its role in sleep regulation, melatonin's antioxidant properties further enhance its neuroprotective effects, making it a key supplement for those looking to improve brain health and longevity.

Margaret's case demonstrates the transformative potential of high-dose melatonin for individuals at risk of cognitive decline. By restoring her sleep and supporting her brain's detox pathways, Margaret was able to slow the progression of dementia and improve her quality of life. For anyone experiencing sleep disturbances or early signs of cognitive impairment, melatonin offers a safe, effective way to enhance brain function and protect against long-term neurodegeneration.

Vitamin D: A Key Player in Preventing Cognitive Decline

Vitamin D's Role in Amyloid-Beta Clearance

Vitamin D is widely recognised for its role in supporting bone health and immune function, but its importance extends far beyond these well-known benefits. Recent research highlights Vitamin D's **neuroprotective properties**, particularly its role in maintaining **cognitive health** and preventing neurodegenerative diseases like **Alzheimer's disease**. One of the key ways Vitamin D protects the brain is by promoting the clearance of **amyloid-beta,** a toxic protein that contributes to the formation of plaques in the brain, a hallmark of Alzheimer's.

Amyloid-beta is produced as a byproduct of normal brain activity, but when it accumulates in excess, it forms sticky plaques between neurons, disrupting cell-to-cell communication and triggering **neuroinflammation**. Over time, these plaques contribute to the progressive cognitive decline seen in Alzheimer's disease. The body has mechanisms to clear amyloid-beta, particularly through the **glymphatic system,** but these pathways can become impaired due to ageing, poor sleep, or nutrient deficiencies—especially Vitamin D deficiency.

Vitamin D acts through several pathways to protect the brain and enhance the clearance of amyloid-beta. One of its primary roles is regulating **calcium homeostasis** in neurons. Proper calcium signalling is essential for neuron function, and imbalances can lead to **oxidative stress**, mitochondrial dysfunction, and ultimately neuronal death. Vitamin D helps prevent these imbalances, reducing neuronal vulnerability to damage caused by amyloid-beta plaques.

Additionally, Vitamin D stimulates the production of **antimicrobial peptides** such as **cathelicidin** and **defensins,** which are involved in protecting the brain from infection and inflammation. These peptides enhance the brain's immune response, helping microglial cells—the brain's resident immune cells—more effectively clear amyloid-beta and other toxic proteins. By reducing inflammation and promoting the removal of amyloid-beta, Vitamin D plays a key role in maintaining cognitive function and preventing the buildup of plaques that lead to Alzheimer's disease.

Vitamin D's **anti-inflammatory effects** also contribute to its neuroprotective properties. Chronic **neuroinflammation** is a significant factor in cognitive decline, and Vitamin D helps modulate the brain's immune response by suppressing the release of **pro-inflammatory cytokines**. This reduction in inflammation not only protects neurons but also improves the brain's ability to detoxify and repair itself, reducing the risk of neurodegeneration.

Despite its critical role in brain health, **Vitamin D deficiency** is widespread, particularly among older adults. As people age, their skin's ability to synthesise Vitamin D from sunlight decreases, and they may spend less time outdoors, further contributing to low levels of this important nutrient. Studies show that individuals with lower levels of Vitamin D are more likely to experience **cognitive decline** and are at a greater risk of developing **Alzheimer's disease**. Ensuring adequate Vitamin D levels through sun exposure, diet, or supplementation is therefore essential for preserving cognitive health and preventing the accumulation of toxic proteins in the brain.

Case Study: Reversing Cognitive Decline with Vitamin D Supplementation

Patient Profile:

- **Name**: Harold, age 68
- **Occupation**: Retired architect
- **Symptoms**: Increasing forgetfulness, difficulty concentrating, confusion with familiar tasks
- **Background**: Harold had been experiencing memory problems for about two years. He would often forget

recent conversations, misplace everyday objects like keys, and struggle to follow through with familiar tasks like balancing his chequebook or preparing meals. His cognitive decline was subtle at first, but gradually became more noticeable, especially to his family. Harold had a history of **Vitamin D deficiency**, which had been diagnosed several years earlier, but he had not consistently taken supplements.

Clinical Findings:

- **Cognitive assessments** showed a decline in **short-term memory, executive function**, and **attention**—areas often affected in the early stages of cognitive decline.
- **Blood tests** revealed that Harold's Vitamin D levels were critically low, with a serum level of **17 ng/mL**, well below the optimal range of **30-50 ng/mL**.
- **Neuroimaging** indicated a moderate accumulation of **amyloid-beta plaques** in the brain, particularly in the hippocampus, the region responsible for memory formation.
- Harold's diet was lacking in Vitamin D-rich foods, and his lifestyle involved limited outdoor activity, further contributing to his deficiency.

Analysis:

Harold's case was indicative of **early-stage cognitive decline**, likely driven by his long-term Vitamin D deficiency and the associated buildup of amyloid-beta plaques. His reduced ability to clear these toxic proteins was leading to memory loss and impaired cognitive function. Given the critical role that Vitamin D plays in both **neuronal health** and **amyloid-beta clearance**, it was clear that correcting his deficiency would be essential in slowing or even reversing his cognitive decline.

Intervention:

Harold's treatment plan focused on restoring his Vitamin D levels to within the optimal range to enhance brain detox and support cognitive function. The key components of his intervention included:

1. **High-Dose Vitamin D Supplementation**: Harold was prescribed **5,000 IU of Vitamin D3** daily to rapidly increase his serum Vitamin D levels. Given his significant deficiency, this higher dose was necessary to restore his levels within a few months. After reaching optimal levels, the dose would be reduced to a maintenance level of **2,000 IU daily**.

2. **Dietary Adjustments**: To further support his Vitamin D levels, Harold incorporated more **Vitamin D-rich foods** into his diet, including fatty fish (such as salmon and sardines), fortified dairy products, and eggs. He also began using a Vitamin D-fortified plant-based milk to enhance his intake.

3. **Sunlight Exposure**: Harold was encouraged to spend **30 minutes outside in direct sunlight** several times a week, particularly during midday when UVB rays are most effective at stimulating Vitamin D production. To ensure maximum benefit, he avoided sunscreen during these short periods of exposure.

4. **Physical Activity**: Harold added regular **walking and light resistance exercises** to his routine, which not only helped improve his overall health but also boosted his **mood** and **mental clarity**. Physical activity has been shown to enhance **cognitive function** and support brain detoxification processes.

5. **Cognitive Stimulation**: To further stimulate his brain and improve neuroplasticity, Harold began engaging in **cognitive exercises**, such as puzzles, memory games, and tasks that challenged his executive function. This brain-training approach was designed to strengthen neural connections and complement the neuroprotective effects of Vitamin D.

Outcome:

After three months of consistent Vitamin D supplementation and lifestyle adjustments, Harold's Vitamin D levels increased to **40 ng/mL**, bringing him within the optimal range for cognitive health. His cognitive performance showed notable improvements, with better memory recall and a reduction in the confusion he had been experiencing with daily tasks. He reported feeling more mentally alert, with less frequent memory lapses.

Follow-up cognitive assessments revealed improvements in Harold's **executive function** and **attention**, and his family noticed a significant positive change in his ability to engage in conversations and manage household tasks. Importantly, a second neuroimaging scan showed a reduction in amyloid-beta plaques in the hippocampus, indicating that his brain was better able to clear toxic proteins as a result of improved Vitamin D levels.

Harold continued on a maintenance dose of Vitamin D and incorporated more outdoor activities into his routine. His cognitive decline had not only stabilised but showed signs of reversal, highlighting the powerful role that **Vitamin D** plays in brain detoxification and cognitive health.

Conclusion

Vitamin D is a critical nutrient for brain health, particularly in its ability to promote the clearance of **amyloid-beta** and protect against cognitive decline. As seen in Harold's case, correcting a Vitamin D deficiency through supplementation and lifestyle adjustments can have a profound impact on both **cognitive function** and **brain detoxification**. For individuals at risk of or already experiencing cognitive decline, ensuring adequate Vitamin D levels is essential for preventing the accumulation of toxic proteins in the brain and reducing the risk of neurodegenerative diseases.

The neuroprotective effects of Vitamin D, combined with its anti-inflammatory and detoxifying properties, make it a powerful tool in the fight against Alzheimer's and other forms of dementia. By maintaining optimal Vitamin D levels through sun exposure, diet, and supplementation, individuals can protect their brains from long-term damage and support cognitive longevity

NAD+ and Procaine: Enhancing Detox Through Cellular Regeneration

NAD+ as an Anti-Ageing Molecule

NAD+ (Nicotinamide Adenine Dinucleotide) is a critical coenzyme found in all living cells, essential for numerous metabolic processes, including **cellular energy production, DNA repair**, and **oxidative stress management**. As we age, NAD+ levels naturally decline, leading to a decrease in mitochondrial efficiency, increased cellular damage, and impaired detoxification. This decline in NAD+ is considered a major contributor to the **ageing process** and age-related diseases, including **cognitive decline** and **neurodegeneration**.

NAD+ plays a vital role in activating **sirtuins**, a family of proteins that regulate cellular health, ageing, and metabolic processes. **SIRT1**, in particular, is crucial for maintaining mitochondrial function and promoting **autophagy**, the process by which cells remove damaged components and toxic waste, including **amyloid-beta** and **tau proteins** that accumulate in the brain and contribute to **Alzheimer's disease**.

As a key molecule in cellular energy production, NAD+ supports the mitochondria—the "powerhouses" of the cell—in generating **ATP (adenosine triphosphate)**, the energy currency of the cell. Mitochondria are especially important in brain cells (neurons), which are highly energy-dependent. When NAD+ levels decline with age, mitochondrial function decreases, leading to an increase in **oxidative stress** and the accumulation of toxic waste in cells, including the brain.

NAD+ is also central to the **DNA repair** process. Throughout life, DNA within cells is constantly being damaged by factors such as oxidative stress, environmental toxins, and UV radiation. **PARPs (Poly ADP-Ribose Polymerases)**, a family of enzymes that repair DNA damage, rely on NAD+ as a fuel source to carry out this repair process. Without sufficient NAD+, DNA damage accumulates, leading to cellular dysfunction and ageing. In the brain, impaired DNA repair can result in neuronal damage and cognitive decline.

By restoring NAD+ levels through supplementation or **NAD+ infusions**, we can support mitochondrial function, enhance cellular detoxification, and promote the repair of DNA. This not only slows the ageing process but also helps **reverse age-related cognitive decline** and protect against neurodegenerative diseases.

Studies have shown that NAD+ supplementation can improve **cognitive function**, boost **memory**, and enhance **mental clarity**, particularly in older adults. NAD+ helps the brain clear out toxic proteins more efficiently, improves synaptic communication between neurons, and promotes **neuroplasticity**—the brain's ability to form new neural connections, which is critical for learning and memory.

Procaine as a Regenerative Biohack

Procaine, traditionally used as a local anaesthetic, has garnered attention for its regenerative properties, particularly in **bioregulatory medicine**. It is used in **anti-ageing protocols** for its ability to **improve cellular communication**, enhance **DNA repair**, and reduce oxidative stress. Procaine has also been studied for its role in improving **circulation**, stimulating **nerve regeneration**, and protecting the brain from the damaging effects of ageing.

Procaine has been found to stabilise cell membranes, protect cells from oxidative damage, and improve the function of **mitochondria**, much like NAD+. By improving mitochondrial function and reducing free radical damage, procaine enhances the brain's ability to detoxify and regenerate. It promotes **cellular repair** and supports **neuronal health,** making it particularly valuable in anti-ageing treatments and cognitive health protocols.

One of the primary mechanisms through which procaine exerts its regenerative effects is by increasing the efficiency of **cellular detox pathways**. By stabilising the cellular environment, procaine allows cells to remove waste products and toxins more effectively. This process is especially important in the brain, where the accumulation of toxic proteins like amyloid-beta and tau contributes to cognitive decline and neurodegeneration.

Procaine is commonly used in **neural therapy,** a bioregulatory treatment that involves injecting small amounts of procaine into specific points of the body to reset the autonomic nervous system and promote healing. This therapy has been used to treat chronic pain, reduce inflammation, and improve **cognitive function.** When used alongside NAD+, procaine acts as a synergistic agent, further enhancing cellular regeneration, detoxification, and brain health.

Case Study: NAD+ and Procaine Reversing Brain Ageing

Patient Profile:

- **Name:** Robert, age 74
- **Occupation:** Retired physician
- **Symptoms**: Cognitive decline, memory loss, mental fatigue, difficulty concentrating
- **Background:** Robert had always prided himself on his sharp mind and ability to problem-solve, but in recent years, he noticed a gradual decline in his cognitive abilities. He frequently forgot conversations, misplaced items, and struggled to focus on complex tasks that once came easily to him. Robert also reported feeling mentally exhausted after short periods of concentration. He had a family history of **Alzheimer's disease,** which heightened his concerns about his cognitive health. In addition, Robert

experienced chronic stress and poor sleep, further contributing to his mental fatigue.

Clinical Findings:

- **Cognitive testing** showed impairments in **working memory, executive function**, and **processing speed**, consistent with early-stage cognitive decline.
- **Blood tests** revealed low levels of **NAD+** and elevated markers of **oxidative stress**, indicating that his cellular repair mechanisms were impaired.
- **Neuroimaging** showed early signs of brain atrophy, particularly in the **hippocampus**, which is critical for memory formation.
- Robert also had **poor sleep quality**, with limited time spent in **deep sleep**, a critical phase for brain detoxification and repair.

Analysis:

Robert's cognitive decline was driven by a combination of factors, including **low NAD+ levels**, mitochondrial dysfunction, oxidative stress, and reduced brain detoxification during sleep. His family history of Alzheimer's and the presence of early signs of brain atrophy further underscored the need for an aggressive intervention to protect his brain from further degeneration. Given his profile, a combined treatment approach using **NAD+ infusions** and **procaine therapy** was recommended to restore cellular health, promote brain detox, and slow cognitive decline.

Intervention:

Robert's treatment plan focused on restoring his NAD+ levels and improving mitochondrial function with a combination of **NAD+ infusions** and **procaine therapy**. The key components of his intervention included:

1. **NAD+ Infusions**: Robert underwent a course of **bi-weekly NAD+ infusions** over eight weeks. The goal was to restore his cellular NAD+ levels, boost mitochondrial function, and

enhance brain detoxification. NAD+ supplementation helps promote autophagy, allowing the brain to clear out toxic proteins more efficiently, and enhances DNA repair to protect neurons from damage.

2. **Procaine Injections**: To complement the NAD+ infusions, Robert received **procaine injections** as part of a **neural therapy** protocol. Small amounts of procaine were injected into specific points to improve cellular communication, reduce oxidative stress, and stimulate nerve regeneration. The procaine injections also helped modulate his autonomic nervous system, reducing his chronic stress levels and improving his sleep quality.

3. **Lifestyle Modifications**: Robert was advised to improve his sleep hygiene by following a consistent bedtime routine, limiting blue light exposure before bed, and engaging in relaxation techniques such as **mindfulness meditation**. These practices were designed to improve his sleep quality and enhance the brain's natural detoxification processes during the night.

4. **Dietary Adjustments**: Robert's diet was adjusted to include more **antioxidant-rich foods** like berries, leafy greens, and nuts, as well as **omega-3 fatty acids** from fish and flaxseeds to support brain health and reduce inflammation. He also incorporated **resveratrol supplements**, a compound known to activate sirtuins and mimic the effects of NAD+ on cellular longevity.

5. **Exercise Routine**: To further boost mitochondrial function and cognitive health, Robert began a regular **exercise regimen** that included **aerobic exercise** and **resistance training**. Exercise has been shown to increase NAD+ levels naturally and promote the release of growth factors that support neuroplasticity and cognitive function.

Outcome:

After eight weeks of NAD+ infusions and procaine therapy, Robert reported significant improvements in his cognitive function and overall energy levels. His mental clarity had returned, and he no longer felt mentally fatigued after short periods of concentration. His memory improved, and he was able to engage in complex tasks with greater focus and ease. Follow-up cognitive testing showed improvements in **executive function**, **working memory**, and **processing speed**, indicating that his cognitive decline had stabilised.

Neuroimaging conducted three months after the treatment revealed a slowing of brain atrophy, particularly in the hippocampus, suggesting that the combined NAD+ and procaine therapy had helped protect against further neuronal damage. Robert's **sleep quality** also improved, with more time spent in **deep non-REM sleep**, allowing his brain to detoxify more effectively during the night.

Overall, Robert's cognitive health had significantly improved, and he continued to receive **maintenance NAD+ infusions** every three months to preserve his gains and protect his brain from further ageing.

While procaine acts as a **regenerative biohack**, improving cellular communication, reducing oxidative stress, and promoting nerve regeneration. Together, NAD+ and procaine form a synergistic approach to reversing the effects of brain ageing by enhancing mitochondrial function, clearing out toxic proteins, and supporting the repair and regeneration of neurons.

Conclusion

The case of Robert illustrates the profound impact that these two therapies can have on cognitive health. By combining **NAD+ infusions** with **procaine therapy**, it is possible to not only slow cognitive decline but also reverse some of the effects of brain ageing, offering hope for individuals experiencing early signs of neurodegeneration. As research into NAD+ and procaine continues to evolve, these therapies hold the promise of revolutionising how we approach brain health and ageing, offering a way to maintain cognitive vitality well into old age.

CoQ10: Mitochondrial Powerhouse for Brain Health

CoQ10's Role in Brain Detox and Mitochondrial Health

Coenzyme Q10 (CoQ10) is a naturally occurring compound found in every cell of the body, where it plays a critical role in energy production and **mitochondrial function**. The mitochondria, often referred to as the "powerhouses" of the cell, are responsible for generating energy in the form of **ATP (adenosine triphosphate)**, which is necessary for all cellular functions. CoQ10 is a key component of the mitochondrial electron transport chain, where it facilitates the conversion of nutrients into ATP, making it essential for **cellular energy metabolism**.

In addition to its role in energy production, CoQ10 acts as a **powerful antioxidant**, protecting cells, including neurons, from damage caused by **oxidative stress**. Oxidative stress occurs when there is an imbalance between free radicals (unstable molecules) and antioxidants, leading to cell damage. In the brain, oxidative stress is a major contributor to **neurodegeneration**, as it damages neurons, disrupts synaptic communication, and impairs the brain's ability to detoxify. By neutralising free radicals, CoQ10 helps protect the brain from oxidative damage and supports its detoxification processes.

As we age, the body's natural levels of CoQ10 decline, leading to reduced mitochondrial efficiency, increased oxidative stress, and greater vulnerability to **cognitive decline**. Low levels of CoQ10 have been associated with a range of neurodegenerative diseases, including **Alzheimer's disease**, **Parkinson's disease**, and **Huntington's disease**. The decline in CoQ10 levels affects the brain's ability to detoxify itself from harmful proteins like **amyloid-beta** and **tau**, which are known to accumulate in neurodegenerative conditions.

In the context of **brain detox**, CoQ10 plays a vital role in maintaining mitochondrial health, which is essential for the brain's energy demands. Neurons require a tremendous amount of energy to function properly, and when mitochondrial function declines, brain cells are less efficient at removing toxic waste products. This can lead to the buildup of harmful proteins and oxidative byproducts, which contribute to the development of cognitive impairments and neurodegenerative diseases.

CoQ10 supplementation has been shown to improve **mitochondrial function**, reduce oxidative stress, and enhance the brain's ability to clear out toxic proteins. In particular, CoQ10 supports the **glymphatic system**, the brain's waste clearance mechanism, by boosting mitochondrial energy production during sleep, when the glymphatic system is most active. This enhanced clearance of metabolic waste helps protect neurons and preserves cognitive function, especially in ageing individuals.

Research has demonstrated that CoQ10 supplementation can slow the progression of neurodegenerative diseases by improving energy metabolism in the brain and reducing oxidative damage. In individuals with **mild cognitive impairment (MCI)** or early-stage Alzheimer's disease, CoQ10 has been shown to enhance memory, attention, and mental clarity, making it a valuable supplement for those looking to maintain cognitive health and prevent cognitive decline.

Case Study: CoQ10 Infusions and Cognitive Performance

Patient Profile:

- **Name**: Susan, age 65
- **Occupation**: Retired school principal
- **Symptoms**: Mild cognitive impairment, mental fatigue, forgetfulness, difficulty concentrating
- **Background**: Over the past two years, Susan had noticed subtle but persistent declines in her cognitive abilities. She often struggled to recall names, forgot where she placed

things, and found it harder to concentrate during conversations or tasks that required focus. Susan also experienced frequent **mental fatigue**, particularly in the afternoon, and felt that her energy levels had decreased since retirement. She had no family history of Alzheimer's disease but was concerned about her cognitive health as she aged. Her diet and exercise habits were generally healthy, but she did not take any supplements regularly.

Clinical Findings:

- Cognitive assessments showed early signs of mild cognitive impairment (MCI), with specific deficits in short-term memory and attention span.
- Blood tests revealed **low levels of CoQ10** and elevated **oxidative stress markers**, indicating mitochondrial dysfunction and increased vulnerability to cognitive decline.
- **Neuroimaging** indicated minor reductions in brain volume, particularly in the **hippocampus**, a region associated with memory formation.
- Susan's energy levels were below average for her age, likely due to reduced mitochondrial efficiency.

Analysis:

Susan's cognitive decline appeared to be linked to a combination of factors, including mitochondrial dysfunction, oxidative stress, and age-related reductions in CoQ10 levels. The low levels of CoQ10 were impairing her brain's ability to efficiently produce energy and detoxify itself from oxidative damage, contributing to her memory problems and mental fatigue. Given her mild cognitive impairment, early intervention with CoQ10 supplementation and **CoQ10 infusions** was recommended to improve mitochondrial function, enhance brain detoxification, and support cognitive performance.

Intervention:

Susan's treatment plan focused on restoring her CoQ10 levels and optimising mitochondrial function through a combination of **CoQ10 oral supplementation** and **CoQ10 intravenous infusions**. The key components of her intervention included:

1. **CoQ10 Infusions**: Susan received weekly **CoQ10 infusions** for six weeks to rapidly increase her CoQ10 levels and support mitochondrial function. The intravenous delivery method ensured that high doses of CoQ10 reached her brain cells, where it was needed most. These infusions aimed to enhance her brain's energy production and improve the clearance of oxidative byproducts.

2. **Oral CoQ10 Supplementation**: In addition to the infusions, Susan was prescribed a daily **CoQ10 supplement** (300 mg) to maintain elevated levels of CoQ10 in her body. This oral supplementation would help support her brain's energy needs and reduce oxidative stress over the long term.

3. **Dietary Adjustments**: Susan's diet was adjusted to include more **antioxidant-rich foods** such as berries, dark leafy greens, and nuts to further reduce oxidative stress and support brain detoxification. Foods rich in **healthy fats**, such as avocados and salmon, were also included to enhance mitochondrial function and energy production.

4. **Exercise Regimen**: Susan began a moderate **exercise routine** that included both aerobic exercise (walking, swimming) and resistance training. Exercise has been shown to increase CoQ10 levels naturally and improve mitochondrial efficiency, which was essential for maintaining her energy levels and cognitive health.

5. **Sleep Optimisation**: Because the glymphatic system is most active during deep sleep, Susan was encouraged to improve her **sleep hygiene** by maintaining a consistent bedtime, limiting screen time before bed, and creating a restful sleep environment. Better sleep would allow her brain to detoxify more effectively during the night.

Outcome:

After completing the six-week course of CoQ10 infusions, Susan reported significant improvements in her cognitive function and energy levels. She experienced fewer memory lapses, felt more mentally alert throughout the day, and was able to focus on tasks for longer periods without fatigue. Her cognitive assessments showed modest improvements in **short-term memory** and **attention span**, indicating that her mild cognitive impairment had stabilised.

Follow-up blood tests revealed that her **CoQ10 levels** had returned to within the optimal range, and her oxidative stress markers had decreased, suggesting that her mitochondrial function had improved. Susan's neuroimaging results also showed no further reduction in hippocampal volume, indicating that her brain health had been preserved.

Susan continued with a maintenance dose of CoQ10 supplementation and remained physically active to support her mitochondrial health. She reported feeling more energised and mentally clear, and her cognitive performance remained stable at subsequent follow-up appointments.

Conclusion

CoQ10 is a vital nutrient for brain health, particularly in its ability to support mitochondrial function, reduce oxidative stress, and promote brain detoxification. As we age, declining CoQ10 levels impair the brain's ability to produce energy and clear out toxic proteins, contributing to cognitive decline and an increased risk of neurodegenerative diseases. Supplementing with CoQ10, either through oral supplements or intravenous infusions, can help restore mitochondrial function, enhance brain detox, and improve cognitive performance.

Susan's case demonstrates the powerful impact of CoQ10 on cognitive health, particularly in ageing individuals experiencing early signs of cognitive decline. By restoring her CoQ10 levels, improving mitochondrial efficiency, and reducing oxidative stress, Susan was able to stabilise her cognitive function and regain her mental clarity. CoQ10 offers a promising intervention for those looking to protect their brain health, slow cognitive decline, and maintain cognitive vitality as they age.

Peptides as Bioregulators: Enhancing Brain Detox and Cognitive Function

Cerebrolysin, Semax, Dihexa, and Other Key Peptides

Peptides are short chains of amino acids that act as **bioregulators**, influencing various physiological processes in the body. In recent years, peptides have gained attention for their potential in **neuroprotection**, **brain detoxification**, and **cognitive enhancement**. Unlike traditional pharmaceuticals, peptides are highly specific in their action and can regulate critical pathways involved in **neuroplasticity**, **neuroinflammation**, and **cellular detoxification**. This makes them an attractive option for individuals looking to optimise brain health and slow cognitive decline.

Several peptides have shown promise in enhancing **brain detox** and supporting cognitive function. Among the most well-researched are **Cerebrolysin, Semax, Dihexa, GHK-Cu**, and **Thymosin Beta-4**, each of which offers unique benefits for brain health. These peptides promote neuronal repair, reduce neuroinflammation, and support the clearance of toxic proteins such as **amyloid-beta** and **tau**, both of which contribute to neurodegenerative diseases like **Alzheimer's**.

Cerebrolysin: The Neurorestorative Peptide

Cerebrolysin is a peptide complex derived from porcine brain tissue that contains neurotrophic factors and amino acids, which are essential for **neuronal repair** and **neuroprotection**. It has been extensively studied for its ability to enhance **cognitive function**, support brain detox, and protect against **neurodegenerative**

diseases. Cerebrolysin acts by mimicking the activity of **neurotrophic factors**, such as **nerve growth factor (NGF)** and **brain-derived neurotrophic factor (BDNF)**, which promote neuronal survival and the formation of new neural connections.

One of Cerebrolysin's key benefits is its ability to reduce **neuroinflammation** and promote the clearance of toxic proteins like **amyloid-beta**. In individuals with **mild cognitive impairment (MCI)** and **Alzheimer's disease**, Cerebrolysin has been shown to improve **memory, attention**, and **executive function**. It also stimulates **synaptic plasticity**, which is crucial for learning and memory retention.

Moreover, Cerebrolysin has **antioxidant properties**, reducing oxidative damage in the brain and supporting mitochondrial function, both of which are essential for maintaining cognitive health and promoting brain detox. Clinical trials have demonstrated that Cerebrolysin can slow the progression of Alzheimer's and other forms of dementia, making it a powerful tool for **neuroprotection**.

Semax: The Cognitive Enhancer

Semax is a synthetic peptide derived from **adrenocorticotropic hormone (ACTH)**, but it does not have the hormonal effects of ACTH. Instead, it acts as a potent **cognitive enhancer** and **neuroprotector**. Semax is primarily known for its ability to improve **focus, memory**, and **mental clarity** by increasing the levels of **BDNF** in the brain. BDNF is critical for supporting **neurogenesis**—the growth of new neurons—and for strengthening synaptic connections between neurons.

Semax also has **anti-inflammatory** and **antioxidant** properties, making it effective in reducing oxidative stress and neuroinflammation, which are common in ageing and neurodegenerative diseases. By reducing neuroinflammation, Semax helps improve brain detoxification processes, supporting the clearance of harmful proteins and waste products that accumulate in the brain over time.

In addition to its cognitive-enhancing effects, Semax is used to treat **ischemic stroke**, where it promotes the recovery of brain function by enhancing blood flow to the brain and supporting neuronal repair. Its ability to increase **cerebral circulation** also makes it a valuable tool for individuals experiencing brain fog, mental fatigue, or cognitive decline related to poor blood flow.

Dihexa: The Neuroplasticity Activator

Dihexa is a synthetic peptide that has gained attention for its remarkable ability to enhance **synaptogenesis**—the formation of new synapses in the brain. Synaptogenesis is critical for **neuroplasticity**, which allows the brain to adapt, learn new information, and recover from injury. Dihexa is often referred to as a **"neuroplasticity activator"** due to its potency in promoting synaptic growth and strengthening neural connections.

What makes Dihexa unique is its ability to **cross the blood-brain barrier** easily, allowing it to exert its effects directly on brain tissue. This peptide specifically targets the formation of new synapses, which is essential for learning, memory retention, and cognitive flexibility. Dihexa has been shown to improve cognitive function in models of **Alzheimer's disease**, **traumatic brain injury**, and other neurodegenerative conditions.

Dihexa's impact on **neuroplasticity** also makes it valuable for enhancing **brain detoxification**. By promoting the growth of new neural connections, Dihexa helps the brain recover from damage and improves its ability to clear out toxic proteins and other metabolic waste. This process is particularly important for individuals at risk of neurodegenerative diseases, as the brain's natural detox pathways become less efficient with age.

GHK-Cu: The Anti-Ageing Peptide

GHK-Cu is a copper-binding peptide that is known for its powerful **anti-ageing** and **tissue-regenerative** properties. While GHK-Cu is most commonly used in **skin regeneration** and wound healing, recent research has highlighted its benefits for **brain health**. GHK-Cu has **anti-inflammatory, antioxidant**, and **neuroprotective** effects, making it a valuable tool for preventing cognitive decline and supporting brain detoxification.

In the brain, GHK-Cu promotes the **expression of genes** related to neuronal health, reducing neuroinflammation, and enhancing synaptic plasticity. It also supports the repair of **DNA damage**, which is critical for preventing the accumulation of toxic proteins and maintaining cellular health. By promoting gene expression related to **cellular repair** and **detoxification**, GHK-Cu helps protect the brain from oxidative stress and the effects of ageing.

Additionally, GHK-Cu has been shown to stimulate **stem cell activity**, supporting the regeneration of damaged neurons and improving cognitive function in ageing individuals. Its ability to reduce inflammation and enhance mitochondrial function makes it an excellent candidate for individuals looking to optimise brain detox and prevent neurodegeneration.

Thymosin Beta-4: The Repair Peptide

Thymosin Beta-4 (TB-4) is a naturally occurring peptide involved in **tissue repair** and **cellular regeneration**. In the context of brain health, TB-4 is known for its ability to promote **neuroregeneration** and **reduce inflammation**. It plays a critical role in repairing damaged tissues, including neurons, by promoting **cell migration**, **angiogenesis** (the formation of new blood vessels), and **cytoskeletal repair**.

Thymosin Beta-4's anti-inflammatory properties make it particularly effective in reducing **neuroinflammation**, which is a key driver of cognitive decline and neurodegenerative diseases. By reducing inflammation in the brain, TB-4 helps improve brain detoxification and supports the clearance of toxic proteins, allowing neurons to function more efficiently.

TB-4 has also been shown to promote **neuroprotection** in models of **traumatic brain injury** and **stroke**, where it helps reduce damage to brain tissue and supports the recovery of cognitive function. Its ability to stimulate cellular repair and regeneration makes it a powerful tool for enhancing **brain detox** and protecting against age-related cognitive decline.

Case Study: Peptide Therapy for Neuroprotection and Detox

Patient Profile:

- **Name:** David, age 60
- **Occupation:** Retired engineer
- **Symptoms:** Memory lapses, difficulty concentrating, mental fatigue, poor cognitive flexibility
- **Background:** David has been experiencing a subtle cognitive decline over the past few years, with increasing difficulty focusing on tasks, recalling recent events, and maintaining mental clarity. He often felt mentally fatigued, especially in the afternoons, and noticed a reduction in his ability to multitask or adapt to new information. David had a family history of **Alzheimer's disease**, which raised concerns about his cognitive health. He sought treatment to improve his brain function and prevent further cognitive decline.

Clinical Findings:

- **Cognitive testing** revealed deficits in **short-term memory, executive function**, and **processing speed**, consistent with early-stage cognitive decline.
- **Blood tests** showed elevated markers of **oxidative stress** and inflammation, likely contributing to his cognitive symptoms.
- **Neuroimaging** revealed minor **atrophy** in the hippocampus, a brain region crucial for memory formation and learning.

- David's overall energy levels were low, and he struggled to maintain mental focus for extended periods.

Analysis:

David's cognitive decline was likely linked to a combination of factors, including **oxidative stress**, **inflammation**, and **mitochondrial dysfunction**. The early signs of hippocampal atrophy and his family history of Alzheimer's disease suggested that early intervention with **peptide therapy** could help protect his brain and support detoxification processes. A combination of peptides targeting neuroplasticity, inflammation reduction, and brain detoxification was recommended to improve his cognitive function and prevent further decline.

Intervention:

David's treatment plan included a combination of **Cerebrolysin**, **Semax**, and **Dihexa** to enhance neuroprotection, promote brain detoxification, and improve cognitive function:

1. **Cerebrolysin Injections**:
   David received **Cerebrolysin** injections twice a week for 10 weeks. The goal was to enhance **neuroplasticity**, promote the growth of new neural connections, and support the brain's detox pathways by mimicking the activity of natural neurotrophic factors. Cerebrolysin's ability to reduce neuroinflammation and protect neurons from oxidative stress was expected to slow the progression of cognitive decline.
2. **Semax Nasal Spray**:
   To improve **focus, memory**, and **mental clarity**, David used **Semax** nasal spray daily. This peptide increased his brain's levels of **BDNF**, which is crucial for cognitive flexibility, learning, and memory retention. Semax also supported **cerebral circulation**, improving blood flow to the brain and helping reduce the effects of mental fatigue and brain fog.
3. **Dihexa Oral Supplementation**:
   David was prescribed **Dihexa** in oral form, taken daily. Dihexa is a potent **neuroplasticity activator** that specifically promotes

synaptogenesis. By enhancing the formation of new synapses, Dihexa helped improve David's ability to adapt to new information, multitask, and recall memories more effectively. Dihexa's neuroprotective properties also helped counteract the early signs of hippocampal atrophy.

4. **GHK-Cu Cream:**

To support **cellular repair** and reduce inflammation, David applied a topical **GHK-Cu peptide cream** to his neck and temples daily. This peptide helped activate genes related to **neuroprotection**, reduced oxidative stress and supported brain detoxification processes. The GHK-Cu cream also aided in maintaining overall brain health by promoting mitochondrial function and reducing neuroinflammation.

5. **Thymosin Beta-4** (TB-4) Injections:

To further enhance **neuroregeneration** and **reduce neuroinflammation**, David received **Thymosin Beta-4** injections once per week for 10 weeks. This peptide promoted the repair of damaged neurons, reduced inflammation in brain tissue, and supported the recovery of cognitive function by encouraging cellular regeneration.

6. **Lifestyle and Diet Optimisation:**

David was encouraged to maintain a **brain-healthy diet,** rich in **omega-3 fatty acids, antioxidants,** and **anti-inflammatory foods** like berries, leafy greens, and fatty fish. In combination with his peptide therapy, these dietary changes supported mitochondrial function and reduced oxidative stress in the brain.

7. **Exercise and Cognitive Training:**

David incorporated a moderate **exercise regimen,** including both **aerobic exercises** and **resistance training,** which have been shown to enhance **BDNF levels** and improve overall brain function. He also engaged in **cognitive training exercises,** such as puzzles, memory games, and reading, to strengthen neural connections and improve cognitive flexibility.

Outcome

After 12 weeks of peptide therapy, David experienced significant improvements in his cognitive function and overall mental clarity. His memory lapses became less frequent, and he reported feeling more focused and mentally sharp throughout the day. His mental fatigue diminished, allowing him to engage in tasks for longer periods without losing concentration.

Follow-up cognitive testing showed improvements in **executive function, working memory**, and **processing speed**, indicating that his cognitive decline had stabilised. Neuroimaging revealed no further hippocampal atrophy, and his **blood markers** for oxidative stress and inflammation had decreased significantly, suggesting that the peptides were effectively supporting **brain detoxification** and reducing cellular damage.

David continued to use **maintenance doses** of **Semax** and **Dihexa**, along with periodic **Cerebrolysin injections**, to preserve his cognitive gains and protect against further cognitive decline. He remained physically active and adhered to his brain-healthy diet, ensuring that his brain remained in optimal condition for years to come.

Conclusion

Peptides such as Cerebrolysin, Semax, Dihexa, GHK-Cu, and Thymosin Beta-4 offer promising avenues for brain detoxification, neuroprotection, and cognitive enhancement. By promoting neuroplasticity, reducing neuroinflammation, and enhancing mitochondrial function, these peptides provide a comprehensive approach to preventing and reversing cognitive decline. David's case illustrates the potential of peptide therapy to stabilise and even improve cognitive function in individuals experiencing early signs of neurodegeneration. As peptide research continues to evolve, these treatments are likely to play a key role in the future of brain health and cognitive longevity.

Managing EMF Exposure: Protecting the Brain from Electromagnetic Stress

The Link Between EMF Exposure and Cognitive Decline

In our increasingly connected world, **electromagnetic fields (EMF)**, emitted from devices like smartphones, Wi-Fi routers, computers, and other electronic devices, have become ubiquitous. While these technologies have transformed our daily lives, the growing concern over the potential negative health impacts of prolonged EMF exposure, particularly on the brain, is a subject of ongoing research.

EMFs are invisible areas of energy, often referred to as **radiation**, which can be classified into two categories: **ionising** and **non-ionising radiation**. Ionising radiation (such as X-rays and gamma rays) has enough energy to remove tightly bound electrons from atoms, which can damage DNA. Non-ionising radiation, such as that emitted by cell phones and Wi-Fi, has less energy but can still affect biological systems over time, particularly with chronic exposure.

Prolonged exposure to **non-ionising EMFs**, particularly those from **radiofrequency (RF)** sources, has been linked to **cognitive decline, sleep disturbances**, and **neuroinflammation**. Studies suggest that EMFs may increase the production of **reactive oxygen species (ROS)**, leading to **oxidative stress** in the brain, which can damage neurons and impair cognitive function. Oxidative stress caused by EMF exposure can result in **mitochondrial dysfunction**, reducing the brain's ability to produce energy efficiently and leading to an accumulation of toxic waste, including **amyloid-beta** and **tau proteins**. These toxic proteins are linked to neurodegenerative diseases such as **Alzheimer's** and **Parkinson's disease**.

One of the key concerns regarding EMF exposure is its potential to disrupt the **blood-brain barrier (BBB)**, a protective layer that prevents harmful substances from entering the brain. Research has shown that prolonged exposure to EMFs can increase the permeability of the BBB, allowing toxins and inflammatory molecules to penetrate the brain more easily. This can lead to **neuroinflammation**, oxidative damage, and an impaired ability to detoxify the brain. Over time, these processes can accelerate cognitive decline, especially in individuals who are already at risk for neurodegenerative diseases.

Furthermore, EMFs can interfere with the brain's natural **electrical activity**, affecting **neural communication** and leading to symptoms such as brain fog, mental fatigue, and difficulty concentrating. Sleep, which is essential for brain detoxification and cognitive restoration, is also impacted by EMF exposure. Studies have shown that exposure to EMFs, particularly at night, can disrupt the production of **melatonin**, the hormone responsible for regulating sleep-wake cycles and promoting deep, restorative sleep. This reduction in melatonin can impair the **glymphatic system**, which is most active during deep sleep and is responsible for clearing waste from the brain, including toxic proteins.

As research continues to investigate the link between EMF exposure and cognitive decline, there is increasing evidence to suggest that reducing EMF exposure may be beneficial for maintaining **brain health** and preventing the onset of **neurodegenerative diseases**.

Case Study: Reducing EMF for Better Brain Health

Patient Profile:

- **Name**: Sarah, age 52
- **Occupation**: Corporate executive
- **Symptoms**: Chronic brain fog, difficulty focusing, poor sleep quality, frequent headaches
- **Background**: Sarah had been experiencing cognitive issues for over a year, with increasing difficulty concentrating at work, remembering important details, and maintaining mental clarity throughout the day. In addition, she suffered from frequent **headaches** and **insomnia**,

often waking up feeling unrefreshed. Despite leading an otherwise healthy lifestyle—exercising regularly and eating a balanced diet—her cognitive symptoms persisted. Sarah worked long hours in a high-stress environment, where she was constantly surrounded by electronic devices such as smartphones, laptops, and Wi-Fi routers. Her office and home were filled with technology, contributing to significant EMF exposure.

Clinical Findings:

- Cognitive assessments revealed impairments in **attention**, **short-term memory**, and **executive function**, consistent with early signs of cognitive decline.
- A **sleep study** showed that Sarah was spending limited time in **deep non-REM sleep**, the phase crucial for brain detoxification and cognitive recovery.
- **Blood tests** indicated elevated levels of **oxidative stress** and **inflammatory markers**, likely linked to chronic EMF exposure.
- A **neuroimaging scan** showed mild brain atrophy, particularly in the **prefrontal cortex**, the region responsible for attention and decision-making, suggesting that her cognitive issues were related to environmental stressors, including EMF exposure.

Analysis:

Sarah's cognitive decline and sleep disturbances were likely exacerbated by her constant exposure to EMFs in both her work and home environments. The frequent use of electronic devices and the presence of multiple sources of **Wi-Fi radiation** in her immediate environment were contributing to **oxidative stress** in her brain, disrupting her sleep and impairing her ability to detoxify and regenerate during the night. Her headaches, brain fog, and mental fatigue were consistent with the symptoms of **electromagnetic hypersensitivity** (EHS), a condition in which individuals are particularly sensitive to EMFs.

Given these findings, it was clear that reducing Sarah's exposure to EMFs and addressing the oxidative stress in her brain would be essential for improving her cognitive function, sleep quality, and overall brain health.

Intervention:

To mitigate the effects of EMF exposure on Sarah's brain and cognitive function, the following intervention plan was implemented:

1. **Creating an EMF-Free Sleep Zone**:
   Sarah was advised to create an **EMF-free environment** in her bedroom to promote better sleep and support brain detox. This involved turning off all electronic devices and **Wi-Fi routers** at night, removing her phone from the bedroom, and using a **battery-operated alarm clock** instead of her smartphone. She also installed **EMF-blocking curtains** and used a **grounding mat** on her bed to reduce electromagnetic radiation while sleeping.

2. **Reducing Daytime EMF Exposure**:
   During the day, Sarah limited her exposure to **Wi-Fi** and electronic devices by using **wired connections** for her computer and avoiding long phone conversations unless using **air tube headsets**, which reduce direct exposure to her brain. She also took regular breaks away from screens and implemented a **20-minute break** after every hour of screen time to reduce mental fatigue and oxidative stress.

3. **Wearing EMF-Blocking Devices**:
   Sarah began wearing **EMF-blocking pendants** and placed **EMF-blocking patches** on her smartphone and laptop to reduce her direct radiation exposure. These devices are designed to shield the body from high levels of EMF, minimising its harmful effects.

4. **Detoxifying with Antioxidants**:
   To address the elevated levels of **oxidative stress** caused by EMF exposure, Sarah was prescribed a high-dose **antioxidant regimen** that included supplements such as **CoQ10, vitamin**

C, **glutathione**, and **alpha-lipoic acid**. These antioxidants helped neutralise free radicals and reduce oxidative damage in her brain, supporting cellular detoxification and mitochondrial function.

5. **Melatonin Supplementation:**

   Given the disruption in Sarah's sleep and **melatonin production** due to EMF exposure, she began taking **melatonin supplements** (5 mg) every night to restore her natural sleep-wake cycle and promote deep, restorative sleep. This helped enhance the activity of her **glymphatic system**, improving brain detoxification during the night.

6. **Mindfulness and Stress Reduction:**

   Since stress can exacerbate the effects of EMF exposure, Sarah incorporated **mindfulness meditation** and **breathing exercises** into her daily routine. This helped reduce her overall stress levels, improve her focus, and enhance her brain's resilience to environmental stressors.

Outcome:

After six weeks of reducing her EMF exposure and implementing the detoxification protocol, Sarah reported significant improvements in her cognitive function and overall well-being. Her **brain fog** and **headaches** had diminished, and she was able to concentrate more effectively at work. She no longer experienced the mental fatigue that had plagued her in the afternoons, and her ability to focus on tasks improved.

Her **sleep quality** improved dramatically, as evidenced by a follow-up sleep study, which showed that she was spending more time in **deep non-REM sleep**. This increase in deep sleep allowed her brain to detoxify more effectively, leading to better mental clarity and memory retention during the day.

Follow-up blood tests revealed a reduction in oxidative stress markers, and her neuroimaging showed no further signs of brain atrophy, indicating that the intervention had successfully protected her brain from further damage. Sarah continued to maintain her low-EMF lifestyle, including wearing EMF-blocking devices and optimising her sleep environment, to preserve her cognitive gains and protect her brain health in the long term.

Conclusion

Electromagnetic fields (EMF), emitted by everyday electronic devices, can have a significant impact on brain health, contributing to cognitive decline, neuroinflammation, and disrupted sleep patterns. Prolonged exposure to EMFs increases **oxidative stress**, damages the **blood-brain barrier**, and impairs the brain's ability to detoxify harmful proteins, accelerating the ageing process and increasing the risk of neurodegenerative diseases.

As Sarah's case illustrates, taking proactive steps to reduce EMF exposure and support brain detox through antioxidant supplementation, improved sleep hygiene, and mindfulness practices can lead to significant improvements in cognitive function and overall brain health. By minimising exposure to electromagnetic stressors and promoting **cellular detoxification**, individuals can protect their brains from the harmful effects of **EMFs**. Reducing EMF exposure not only supports **cognitive performance** but also enhances the brain's ability to detoxify and regenerate, preserving **neuroplasticity** and reducing the risk of cognitive decline.

In an increasingly digital world, where constant exposure to EMFs is inevitable, adopting strategies like **creating EMF-free zones**, using **EMF-blocking devices**, and supporting the body's natural detoxification processes with antioxidants, sleep optimisation, and stress reduction techniques is essential. As more research emerges on the connection between **EMF exposure** and brain health, it becomes clear that taking steps to manage these exposures can have a profound impact on both **cognitive longevity** and **overall well-being**.

Reigniting the Vagus Nerve: Counteracting Sympathetic Drive

The Role of the Vagus Nerve in Detox and Cognitive Function

The **vagus nerve** is one of the most important components of the **parasympathetic nervous system**, often referred to as the **"rest and digest"** system. This nerve acts as a communication superhighway between the brain and various organs, including the heart, lungs, gut, and liver. It plays a key role in regulating essential bodily functions such as heart rate, digestion, and immune response, as well as facilitating the body's ability to **relax, recover,** and **detoxify**. In recent years, research has highlighted the critical role the vagus nerve plays in **cognitive function, emotional regulation,** and **brain detoxification.**

The **vagus nerve** counteracts the **sympathetic nervous system,** which governs the **fight-or-flight response**—a survival mechanism that kicks in during stress. While this response is helpful in short-term, acute situations, chronic stress causes prolonged sympathetic activation, leading to **elevated cortisol levels, increased heart rate,** and **inflammation.** Over time, this continuous sympathetic drive can impair **cognitive function,** increase **neuroinflammation,** and inhibit the brain's natural detox processes. Chronic stress, mediated by the overactivation of the sympathetic nervous system, is a known risk factor for **cognitive decline, memory loss,** and **neurodegenerative diseases** such as **Alzheimer's.**

The **vagus nerve** is a powerful tool for restoring balance, helping to shift the body into a **parasympathetic state,** where **healing** and **recovery** take place. When the vagus nerve is activated, it reduces inflammation by inhibiting the production of **pro-inflammatory cytokines** and promotes the release of **acetylcholine,** a neurotransmitter essential for memory, attention, and learning. By reducing systemic inflammation and promoting **calmness,** the vagus nerve enhances **brain detoxification** by optimising the function of the **glymphatic system**, which is responsible for clearing out toxic proteins like **amyloid-beta** and **tau**.

In addition to its role in **reducing neuroinflammation**, the vagus nerve influences **gut health**, a key factor in brain detox. Known as the **gut-brain axis**, this bidirectional communication between the gut and brain is largely mediated by the vagus nerve. The health of the gut microbiome is crucial for cognitive function and detox, as a healthy gut produces anti-inflammatory compounds like **short-chain fatty acids** that protect the brain. Conversely, an unhealthy gut can lead to **neuroinflammation**, further impairing cognitive performance. Activating the vagus nerve supports a healthy gut environment, which in turn improves cognitive health and enhances the brain's ability to clear toxins.

In modern life, many factors—chronic stress, poor diet, and lack of physical activity—can impair vagal tone (the strength of the vagus nerve's signalling). When a vagal tone is low, the body remains in a prolonged sympathetic state, contributing to systemic inflammation, cognitive dysfunction, and poor detoxification. However, there are several ways to **reignite the vagus nerve** and improve vagal tone, including:

- **Deep breathing exercises**: Slow, diaphragmatic breathing stimulates the vagus nerve, shifting the body into a parasympathetic state.
- **Cold exposure**: Brief cold exposure, such as a cold shower or immersion in cold water, activates the vagus nerve and reduces inflammation.
- **Gargling and singing**: These activities stimulate the muscles at the back of the throat, activating the vagus nerve and promoting relaxation.
- **Mindfulness and meditation**: Mindfulness practices calm the mind and body, reducing sympathetic drive and boosting vagal tone.

- **Vagus nerve stimulation devices**: Devices like the **Sensate** or **gammaCore** offer non-invasive ways to stimulate the vagus nerve through low-level electrical impulses, improving mood, reducing stress, and enhancing brain detoxification.

By incorporating these vagus nerve activation techniques, individuals can reduce chronic stress, improve **cognitive function**, and enhance their brain's ability to detoxify, thus reducing the risk of **neurodegenerative diseases** and promoting overall brain health.

Case Study: Activating the Vagus Nerve to Improve Cognitive Health

Patient Profile:

- **Name**: John, age 58
- **Occupation**: Business executive
- **Symptoms**: Chronic stress, anxiety, mental fatigue, poor memory retention, brain fog
- **Background**: John had been working in a high-stress corporate environment for decades, and over the last few years, he noticed a steady decline in his cognitive abilities. He found it increasingly difficult to focus during meetings, retain information, and make decisions. John experienced frequent **brain fog**, and **mental fatigue**, and often felt overwhelmed. He also suffered from **anxiety** and **poor sleep**, waking up several times during the night and feeling tired in the morning. He relied on caffeine and energy drinks to get through the day, which further disrupted his sleep patterns.

Despite these symptoms, John maintained an overall healthy diet and regular exercise routine but noticed little improvement in his cognitive health. Recognising the potential impact of chronic stress on his brain, John sought help to restore his cognitive function and overall mental clarity.

Clinical Findings:

- Cognitive testing revealed **deficits in working memory**, **focus**, and **processing speed**, consistent with **chronic stress**-related cognitive decline.
- John's heart rate variability (HRV) was low, an indicator of reduced **vagal tone**, suggesting that his **parasympathetic nervous system** was not functioning optimally.
- Blood tests indicated elevated levels of **inflammatory markers**, including **C-reactive protein (CRP)**, a sign of chronic systemic inflammation, likely due to his high-stress levels.
- John's **sleep study** showed fragmented sleep patterns, particularly a lack of **deep non-REM sleep**, a phase essential for brain detox.

Analysis:

John's cognitive decline and brain fog were likely exacerbated by prolonged sympathetic activation and low vagal tone. His body was stuck in a chronic state of **fight-or-flight**, leading to high levels of cortisol, systemic inflammation, and impaired brain detox. Without proper activation of the **vagus nerve**, his body was unable to switch into a parasympathetic state where healing, detoxification, and cognitive recovery could occur. His lack of deep sleep further inhibited the brain's ability to clear out toxic proteins, contributing to his memory issues and mental fatigue.

The goal of his treatment was to **reignite the vagus nerve**, reduce sympathetic drive, and promote a state of relaxation to enhance **brain detoxification** and cognitive function.

Intervention:

John's treatment plan focused on **vagus nerve activation** techniques and stress reduction to improve his cognitive health:

1. **Deep Breathing Exercises**:
   John was taught to practise **deep diaphragmatic breathing** several times a day. He followed a pattern of **4-7-8 breathing**

(inhaling for 4 seconds, holding for 7 seconds, and exhaling for 8 seconds) to stimulate the vagus nerve, lower cortisol levels, and calm his nervous system.

2. **Cold Exposure Therapy:**

   To further activate the vagus nerve, John started taking **cold showers** in the morning. Cold exposure stimulates the vagus nerve by activating the **parasympathetic response**, reducing inflammation and improving stress resilience. After each shower, John reported feeling more awake, clear-headed, and less anxious.

3. **Vagus Nerve Stimulation Device:**

   John began using a **vagus nerve stimulation device** called **Sensate** for 10 minutes each evening. This device applies gentle vibrations to the chest, stimulating the vagus nerve and promoting relaxation. Over time, this helped John reduce his stress levels and improve his sleep quality.

4. **Mindfulness Meditation:**

   John incorporated a daily 15-minute **mindfulness meditation** practice to reduce his overall stress. Meditation calms the mind, reduces sympathetic drive, and enhances vagal tone by encouraging the brain to focus on the present moment, reducing anxiety and mental overload.

5. **Sleep Hygiene and Melatonin:**

   To improve his sleep, John was encouraged to follow a strict **sleep hygiene** routine, which included turning off electronic devices 90 minutes before bed, avoiding caffeine after noon, and using a **blue light filter** on his screens in the evening. He was also prescribed a small dose of **melatonin** (3 mg) to help regulate his sleep-wake cycle and promote deeper sleep, thereby enhancing the brain's detoxification processes.

6. **Anti-Inflammatory Diet:**

   To reduce systemic inflammation, John adopted an **anti-inflammatory diet** rich in omega-3 fatty acids (from fish and flaxseeds), antioxidants (from berries, dark leafy greens, and turmeric), and polyphenols. These dietary changes helped lower his inflammatory markers and supported his cognitive health.

Outcome:

After eight weeks of implementing these vagus nerve activation techniques, John experienced significant improvements in his **cognitive function** and **emotional well-being**. His **brain fog** and **mental fatigue** had diminished, and he felt more focused and clear-headed during the day. He was able to retain information better, concentrate during meetings, and make decisions with greater ease.

John's **sleep quality** also improved, with fewer nighttime awakenings and longer periods of **deep non-REM sleep**. He woke up feeling more refreshed and energised, which contributed to his mental clarity throughout the day. John's **anxiety levels** decreased significantly, and he no longer relied on caffeine or energy drinks to get through the day. His heart rate variability (HRV) improved, indicating a stronger **vagal tone** and blood tests showed a reduction in **inflammatory markers**, including **C-reactive protein (CRP)**, suggesting that the interventions had reduced systemic inflammation.

In follow-up cognitive assessments, John's **working memory**, **focus**, and **processing speed** showed notable improvements, indicating that his brain function had stabilised and even improved. The reduction in chronic stress and the increase in vagal tone allowed his brain to enter a **restorative state**, facilitating better **brain detoxification** and enhancing his cognitive resilience.

John continued with his vagus nerve activation techniques, including deep breathing exercises, cold exposure, and mindfulness meditation, as part of his daily routine. Over time, these practices became integral to maintaining his cognitive health, emotional balance, and overall well-being. He reported feeling more grounded, calm, and mentally sharp, and he felt more capable of handling the demands of his high-stress work environment.

Conclusion

Reigniting the vagus nerve is a powerful tool for counteracting the harmful effects of **chronic sympathetic drive** on brain health. By shifting the body into a **parasympathetic state**, where healing and detoxification occur, vagus nerve activation enhances **cognitive function**, reduces **inflammation**, and improves the brain's ability to clear toxic waste. As John's case illustrates, stimulating the vagus nerve through simple techniques like **deep breathing**, **cold exposure**, and **vagus nerve stimulation devices** can significantly improve cognitive health and emotional well-being.

Incorporating vagus nerve activation into daily life helps mitigate the long-term effects of chronic stress, supports brain detoxification, and promotes **cognitive longevity**, offering a practical approach to maintaining brain health in an increasingly stressful world

Summary: NAD+, Procaine, and CoQ10: Modern Molecules for Neuroprotection

(a)

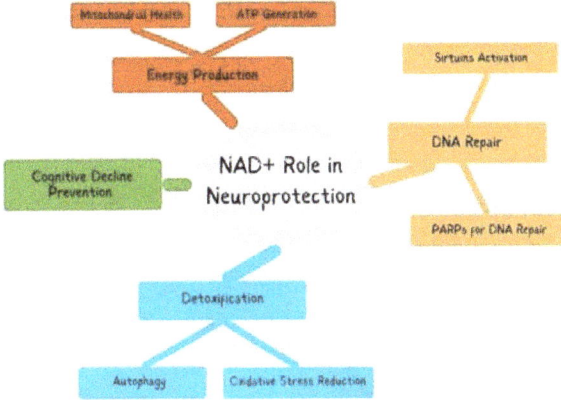

(b)

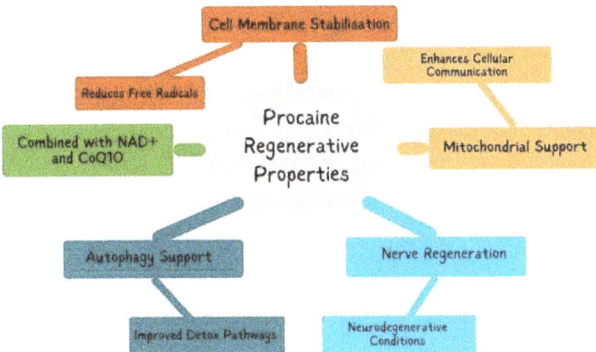

(c)

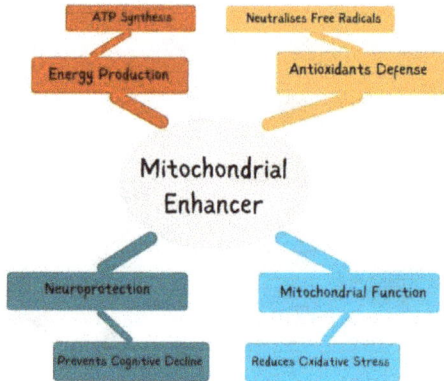

(d)

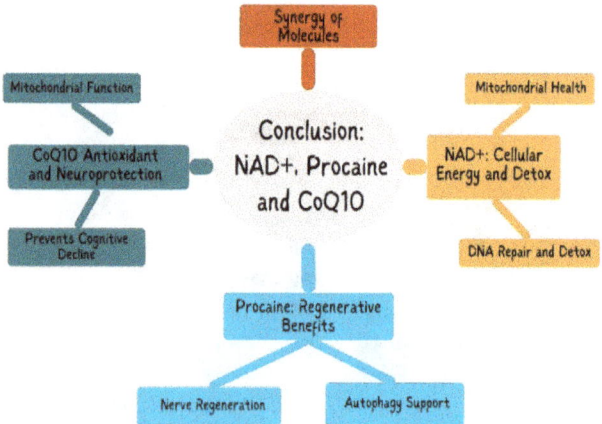

87

Chapter Three: Ancient Practices for Brain Detox: Ayurvedic, Chinese, and Greek Traditions

Ayurvedic Herbs and Practices for Detox

Ayurveda, the ancient medical system originating in India over 5,000 years ago, is one of the oldest approaches to **holistic healing** and places a strong emphasis on **detoxification** (referred to as **Panchakarma**) for maintaining health and longevity. In Ayurveda, brain health is believed to be deeply connected to the balance of the body's **doshas** (Vata, Pitta, and Kapha), and cognitive decline is often seen as a result of imbalances in these fundamental energies, as well as the accumulation of **toxins** (Ama) in the body and mind.

Several **Ayurvedic herbs** are traditionally used to support brain detoxification, protect against cognitive decline, and improve **mental clarity** and **focus**:

1. **Bacopa Monnieri (Brahmi):**
2. Bacopa is one of the most well-known **nootropic herbs** in Ayurveda. It has been used for centuries to enhance memory, support **mental clarity**, and protect the brain from oxidative stress. Modern research confirms Bacopa's role in improving **synaptic communication** in the brain and its ability to promote the clearance of **amyloid-beta**, a protein linked to Alzheimer's disease. Bacopa is also a powerful **antioxidant**, reducing oxidative stress that can impair brain detoxification.
3. **Ashwagandha (Withania Somnifera):**
   Ashwagandha is a key adaptogen in Ayurveda known for its ability to reduce **stress** and **anxiety**, both of which can

negatively affect cognitive health. By lowering **cortisol levels**, Ashwagandha supports the body's ability to enter a parasympathetic state, allowing the brain to detoxify and regenerate more effectively. Additionally, Ashwagandha has **neuroprotective** properties, promoting **nerve regeneration** and reducing **neuroinflammation**.

4. **Gotu Kola (Centella Asiatica):**
   Known as the "**herb of longevity**" in Ayurveda, Gotu Kola has been used to enhance **mental clarity, memory,** and **focus**. It is believed to strengthen the **brain's protective barrier** and reduce neuroinflammation, both of which are critical for effective brain detoxification. Gotu Kola also enhances **circulation to the brain**, improving oxygen and nutrient delivery while promoting the removal of metabolic waste products.

5. **Turmeric (Curcuma Longa):**
   Turmeric, a powerful anti-inflammatory herb, is a staple in Ayurvedic medicine for its ability to combat **oxidative stress** and promote detoxification. The active compound in turmeric, **curcumin,** has been extensively studied for its ability to reduce the accumulation of **amyloid plaques** in the brain, a key feature of neurodegenerative diseases like Alzheimer's. Curcumin also promotes the function of the **glymphatic system**, helping the brain clear out toxic waste products during sleep.

In addition to herbal remedies, Ayurveda incorporates **lifestyle practices** such as **oil pulling, nasya therapy** (herbal oils administered through the nostrils), and **meditation** to promote brain health and support detoxification. **Nasya therapy,** in particular, is used to clear the sinus passages and improve circulation to the brain, helping to enhance cognitive function.

Acupuncture and Traditional Chinese Medicine for Brain Health

Traditional Chinese Medicine (TCM) has a long history of treating cognitive decline and supporting brain detoxification through the use of **herbal medicine, acupuncture**, and **Qigong** (a movement and breathing practice designed to enhance energy flow). TCM views the brain as closely related to the health of the **Kidneys**, which store **Jing**, or essence, believed to be the foundation of vitality and mental sharpness. As we age, this Jing becomes depleted, leading to cognitive decline and memory issues.

Several key **herbs** and practices in TCM are used to support brain health:

1. **Ginkgo Biloba**:
   Ginkgo Biloba is one of the most well-known TCM herbs for supporting **brain health**. It enhances **blood flow to the brain**, improves memory, and reduces **oxidative damage** to neurons. Studies have shown that Ginkgo Biloba can protect against **cognitive decline** by increasing the brain's antioxidant capacity and improving **synaptic plasticity**.
2. **Rehmannia (Shu Di Huang)**:
   Rehmannia is an important herb in TCM used to **nourish the kidneys** and **support Jing**, promoting longevity and brain health. It is often used in formulas designed to treat memory loss and cognitive decline, particularly in older adults. Rehmannia also helps combat **oxidative stress** and supports the **clearance of toxins** from the brain.
3. **Polygala (Yuan Zhi)**:
   Polygala is used in TCM to **calm the mind** and enhance **memory**. It is believed to help resolve emotional blockages, which, according to TCM philosophy, can impair cognitive function. Polygala supports **neuroplasticity** by promoting communication between neurons and enhancing the brain's ability to repair itself.

4. **Acupuncture**:

Acupuncture is a central component of TCM used to **balance energy flow** (Qi) and support the body's natural detox processes. Specific acupuncture points related to brain health, such as **Du 20 (Baihui)**, located at the top of the head, and **GB 20 (Fengchi)**, located at the base of the skull, are often used to **improve cognition** and enhance **circulation** to the brain. By regulating the flow of Qi, acupuncture reduces **inflammation**, lowers **cortisol**, and promotes **mental clarity**.

5. **Qigong**:

This practice combines physical movement, controlled breathing, and mental focus to cultivate **life force energy** (Qi) and support overall health, including brain health. Qigong improves circulation to the brain, reduces stress, and enhances **mind-body** coordination. Regular practice of Qigong can stimulate the brain's detox mechanisms by promoting relaxation and lowering stress-induced inflammation.

Case Study: Ayurvedic Protocols for Cognitive Longevity

Patient Profile:

- **Name**: Priya, age 62
- **Occupation**: Retired teacher
- **Symptoms**: Mild cognitive decline, mental fatigue, occasional memory lapses
- **Background**: Priya had always led a healthy lifestyle, but she began noticing subtle cognitive changes over the past year, including **forgetfulness**, **brain fog**, and difficulty concentrating. She also felt mentally fatigued after performing tasks that required sustained focus. Priya had no family history of neurodegenerative diseases, but she was concerned about her cognitive health as she aged.

Clinical Findings:

- Cognitive assessments revealed **mild deficits in short-term memory** and **mental clarity**, suggesting early-stage cognitive decline.
- Blood tests showed slightly elevated **markers of inflammation**, which can contribute to cognitive impairment over time.
- Priya reported frequent periods of stress due to family responsibilities, which may have exacerbated her cognitive symptoms.

Ayurvedic Intervention:

Priya's treatment plan was based on traditional **Ayurvedic principles** of balancing the **doshas** to restore brain health and detoxify the mind:

1. **Bacopa Monnieri and Ashwagandha:**
    Priya was prescribed a daily combination of **Bacopa Monnieri** and **Ashwagandha** supplements to enhance memory, reduce stress, and support cognitive clarity. The **antioxidant** and **adaptogenic** properties of these herbs were designed to reduce neuroinflammation and support her brain's ability to clear **toxic proteins**.

2. **Turmeric with Black Pepper:**
    To further reduce inflammation, Priya was advised to take **turmeric** (with **black pepper** for better absorption) daily. This combination enhanced her brain's detox pathways by reducing oxidative stress and improving the function of the **glymphatic system**.

3. **Nasya Therapy:**
    To improve **circulation to the brain** and enhance mental clarity, Priya practised **nasya therapy** using **Brahmi oil**. This traditional Ayurvedic practice involved applying a few drops of herbal oil into the nostrils every morning to clear the sinuses and promote brain health.

4. **Mindfulness Meditation**:
   Priya incorporated **mindfulness meditation** into her daily routine to reduce stress and improve mental focus. By promoting relaxation and activating the **vagus nerve**, meditation helped counteract the effects of chronic stress on her brain and supported detoxification.

Outcome:

After three months of following the Ayurvedic protocol, Priya reported significant improvements in her **memory** and **mental clarity**. She felt less mentally fatigued and was able to focus on tasks for longer periods. Cognitive assessments showed that her memory lapses had decreased, and she reported feeling more **balanced** and **focused** overall. Her blood tests showed reduced inflammation markers, indicating that the Ayurvedic herbs and practices had helped **reduce systemic inflammation**, contributing to her cognitive improvements.

Conclusion

Ayurvedic, Chinese, and Greek traditions offer **time-tested practices** for supporting **brain detoxification** and cognitive health. By integrating **herbal medicine, meditation,** and **acupuncture,** these ancient systems provide holistic approaches to **enhancing brain function,** reducing **inflammation,** and promoting the clearance of toxic waste products that contribute.

By integrating **herbal medicine, meditation,** and **acupuncture,** these ancient systems provide holistic approaches to **enhancing brain function,** reducing **inflammation,** and promoting the clearance of toxic waste products that contribute to cognitive decline.

Ayurveda's use of **adaptogenic herbs** like **Ashwagandha** and **Bacopa Monnieri,** combined with detoxification practices like **nasya therapy,** strengthens both the mind and body's ability to cope with stress and clear out toxins. In Traditional Chinese Medicine (TCM), techniques such as **acupuncture** and **Qigong** not only regulate the flow of **Qi** but also optimise brain circulation and detoxification, promoting mental clarity and longevity. By applying these methods, modern individuals can benefit from **natural, non-invasive approaches** to maintaining **cognitive health** and preventing neurodegenerative diseases.

These ancient traditions, backed by modern scientific validation, offer valuable tools for **preventing cognitive decline, enhancing brain detoxification**, and promoting **long-term cognitive longevity**. Whether used as complementary therapies or integrated with modern biohacking techniques, these ancient practices continue to provide profound benefits for brain health in the modern world.

Herbs and Natural Compounds for Brain Detox

Adaptogens, Antioxidants, and Herbal Medicine for Brain Health

Herbs and natural compounds have been used for centuries to support **brain health, enhance cognitive function**, and promote **detoxification**. Modern research has validated many of these traditional remedies, revealing that certain herbs possess powerful **antioxidant** and **anti-inflammatory** properties, while others enhance **neuroplasticity, reduce neuroinflammation**, and support the brain's ability to clear toxic proteins, such as **amyloid-beta** and **tau**, which are implicated in **neurodegenerative diseases**.

Key categories of herbs and compounds that support brain detoxification include **adaptogens, antioxidants**, and other herbal medicines known for their neuroprotective effects. Let's explore some of the most effective herbs in these categories:

Adaptogens for Brain Detox and Cognitive Health

Adaptogens are a class of herbs that help the body adapt to stress, improve resilience, and restore balance to bodily systems. They are particularly valuable for brain detoxification because chronic stress is a major driver of **neuroinflammation** and cognitive decline. Adaptogens work by modulating the release of **stress hormones** like **cortisol**, reducing inflammation, and enhancing the brain's ability to detoxify and repair itself.

1. **Ashwagandha (Withania somnifera)**

   Ashwagandha is one of the most well-known adaptogens in Ayurvedic medicine and has been shown to reduce **cortisol levels**, thereby reducing the chronic stress that impairs cognitive function and brain detox. Ashwagandha promotes **neurogenesis** (the growth of new neurons), enhances **memory**, and protects against neurodegenerative processes by reducing **oxidative stress** in the brain. It also supports the brain's ability to eliminate toxic proteins and enhances **sleep quality**, which is crucial for brain detox.

2. **Rhodiola Rosea**

   Rhodiola is another powerful adaptogen, known for its ability to **reduce mental fatigue**, improve **focus**, and enhance **memory** under stress. It has been shown to increase the brain's capacity to deal with **oxidative stress** and promote **neuroplasticity**, making it an ideal herb for supporting brain detoxification. Rhodiola also boosts **mental clarity** by improving the brain's utilisation of oxygen, which is essential for clearing out metabolic waste products.

3. **Holy Basil (Tulsi)**

   Holy Basil, also known as Tulsi, is revered in Ayurvedic medicine as a powerful **anti-stress** herb that improves **cognitive function**. It has potent **anti-inflammatory** and **antioxidant** properties, reducing brain inflammation and enhancing the body's natural detoxification processes. Holy Basil is also known to **improve mood** and **reduce anxiety**, which are important for maintaining optimal brain health.

Antioxidants for Protecting Brain Cells

Antioxidants are compounds that neutralise **free radicals**, and unstable molecules that can cause oxidative damage to cells, including neurons. The brain is particularly susceptible to oxidative stress because of its high energy demands and oxygen consumption. Antioxidants play a crucial role in protecting neurons from damage, reducing neuroinflammation, and supporting the brain's natural detoxification processes.

1. **Ginkgo Biloba**

   Ginkgo Biloba is a powerful antioxidant that has been used for centuries to enhance **cognitive function** and **memory**. It improves **circulation** to the brain, ensuring that the brain receives adequate oxygen and nutrients while promoting the clearance of toxic waste. Ginkgo's antioxidant properties help protect neurons from oxidative stress and inflammation, both of which contribute to cognitive decline.

2. **Green Tea (Camellia sinensis)**

   Green tea is rich in **catechins**, particularly **epigallocatechin gallate (EGCG)**, which is a potent antioxidant. EGCG has been shown to protect neurons from oxidative damage, reduce neuroinflammation, and promote the clearance of amyloid-beta plaques in the brain. Drinking green tea or taking EGCG supplements can support brain detoxification and reduce the risk of **Alzheimer's disease** and other neurodegenerative conditions.

3. **Resveratrol**

   Resveratrol is a natural compound found in the skin of grapes, blueberries, and other fruits. It is known for its ability to activate **SIRT1**, a protein involved in cellular repair and brain detoxification. Resveratrol also protects neurons from oxidative damage and enhances **mitochondrial function**, ensuring that brain cells have the energy they need to detoxify and regenerate. Research has shown that resveratrol can improve **memory** and **cognitive performance**, particularly in ageing individuals.

4. **Curcumin (Turmeric)**

   Curcumin, the active compound in **turmeric**, is one of the most powerful natural antioxidants and anti-inflammatory agents. It has been shown to reduce **amyloid plaque formation**, protect neurons from oxidative damage, and enhance brain detoxification by supporting the **glymphatic system**, which is responsible for clearing waste from the brain during sleep. Curcumin also enhances **BDNF** levels, promoting **neuroplasticity** and protecting against cognitive decline.

Other Herbal Medicines for Brain Detox

Beyond adaptogens and antioxidants, several other herbs and natural compounds are well-known for their ability to support **brain detoxification, neuroplasticity**, and **cognitive health**.

1. **Lion's Mane Mushroom (Hericium erinaceus)**
   Lion's Mane is a medicinal mushroom known for its ability to stimulate the production of **nerve growth factor (NGF)**, a protein that promotes the growth and repair of neurons. It enhances **synaptic plasticity**, improves memory, and supports brain detox by promoting the clearance of toxic proteins. Studies show that Lion's Mane can reduce symptoms of **mild cognitive impairment (MCI)** and support overall brain health.

2. **Bacopa Monnieri**
   Bacopa, also known as **Brahmi**, is a powerful **nootropic** herb used in Ayurvedic medicine to improve memory and cognitive function. Bacopa enhances **synaptic communication** in the brain, reduces oxidative stress, and supports the brain's natural detox pathways. It is particularly effective in clearing **amyloid-beta**, the protein associated with Alzheimer's disease and has been shown to improve memory retention and learning capacity.

3. **Gotu Kola (Centella Asiatica)**
   Gotu Kola is known for its ability to **improve circulation** to the brain and promote mental clarity. It has been used in traditional medicine for its neuroprotective properties, enhancing **memory, focus**, and **cognitive function**. Gotu Kola also reduces inflammation and promotes **neurogenesis**, helping the brain detoxify and regenerate after injury or during ageing.

Case Study: Herbal Protocols for Cognitive Improvement

Patient Profile:

- **Name:** Elaine, age 67
- **Occupation:** Retired librarian
- **Symptoms:** Memory lapses, mental fatigue, difficulty concentrating
- **Background:** Elaine has been experiencing a subtle cognitive decline over the past two years. She frequently misplaced items, struggled to recall names, and felt mentally fatigued after completing everyday tasks. She also noticed that her ability to focus on reading or solving puzzles had diminished, which concerned her as she had always prided herself on her mental sharpness. Elaine had no significant medical conditions but reported high levels of **stress** and **insomnia**, both of which can impair brain health and detoxification.

Clinical Findings:

- Cognitive assessments revealed mild deficits in **short-term memory, focus,** and **processing speed.**
- Blood tests showed elevated **oxidative stress markers**, which were likely contributing to her cognitive symptoms.
- Elaine's stress levels were high, and she reported poor **sleep quality**, both of which are key contributors to impaired brain detoxification.

Herbal Protocol:

Elaine's treatment plan included a combination of **adaptogens, antioxidants,** and **herbal supplements** to support brain detox, reduce oxidative stress, and improve cognitive function:

1. **Ashwagandha and Rhodiola:**
   Elaine was prescribed a combination of **Ashwagandha** and **Rhodiola** to reduce her stress levels and improve her body's

resilience to chronic stress. These adaptogens helped regulate her **cortisol levels**, enhancing her ability to focus and reducing mental fatigue.

2. **Bacopa Monnieri:**

   To enhance her memory and promote the clearance of toxic proteins, Elaine began taking **Bacopa Monnieri** daily. This nootropic herb supported **synaptic communication** and improved her ability to retain new information.

3. **Lion's Mane Mushroom:**

   Lion's Mane was added to her regimen to stimulate **neurogenesis** and promote the repair of damaged neurons. This medicinal mushroom improved her cognitive performance by enhancing **neuroplasticity** and supporting her brain's detox pathways.

4. **Curcumin with Piperine:**

   To reduce oxidative stress and inflammation in the brain, Elaine was prescribed **curcumin** with **piperine** (black pepper extract) to enhance its absorption. Curcumin's powerful antioxidant effects supported her brain's ability to detoxify and regenerate during sleep.

5. **Green Tea Extract (EGCG):**

   Elaine also incorporated **green tea extract** rich in **EGCG**, a potent antioxidant, to further reduce oxidative stress in her brain and support detoxification. EGCG helped protect her neurons and improve her mental clarity.

Outcome:

After three months of following her herbal protocol, Elaine reported significant improvements in her **memory, mental clarity,** and **ability to focus**. She no longer misplaced items as frequently, found it easier to recall names and could concentrate on reading and solving puzzles without feeling mentally fatigued. Her **cognitive assessments** showed improvements in **short-term memory, focus,** and **processing speed**, indicating that the herbal protocol had effectively supported her brain health.

In addition, her **sleep quality** improved markedly, as she was able to fall asleep more easily and stay asleep throughout the night. This enhancement in sleep not only helped her feel more energised during the day but also promoted her brain's ability to detoxify during deep sleep. Blood tests revealed a reduction in **oxidative stress markers**, suggesting that the adaptogens and antioxidants were effectively reducing inflammation and oxidative damage in her brain.

Elaine also reported feeling **calmer** and more resilient to stress, thanks to the inclusion of **Ashwagandha** and **Rhodiola** in her protocol. These adaptogens helped regulate her cortisol levels, allowing her brain to operate more efficiently and maintain cognitive function without the interference of chronic stress.

Elaine continued with the herbal regimen as part of her long-term cognitive health plan and found that she was able to maintain her improved mental performance and clarity well beyond the initial three-month period. She felt more confident about her cognitive future and attributed much of her progress to the integration of **natural compounds** into her daily routine.

Conclusion

Herbs and natural compounds like **adaptogens**, **antioxidants**, and other **herbal medicines** offer effective, holistic approaches to supporting brain detoxification and enhancing cognitive function. Elaine's case demonstrates how a well-designed herbal protocol can improve memory, reduce oxidative stress, and promote mental clarity, especially when dealing with mild cognitive decline. Incorporating these herbs into a regular wellness routine can help individuals maintain brain health, protect against cognitive decline, and promote long-term **cognitive resilience.**

Fasting and Intermittent Fasting: Ancient Methods for Brain Detox

Fasting, Autophagy, and Brain Detox

Fasting, the practice of abstaining from food for a specified period, is one of the most ancient methods for enhancing health and longevity. Traditionally used in various cultures for spiritual and healing purposes, fasting is now recognised for its profound effects on **brain health**, particularly in the context of **brain detoxification** and **cognitive function**. Recent scientific research has shed light on the mechanisms by which fasting supports **brain detox**, including **autophagy**, **glymphatic system activation**, and the promotion of **neuroplasticity**.

1. Autophagy: The Cellular Detox Mechanism

   Fasting activates a cellular process called **autophagy**, which is essentially the body's way of **self-cleaning**. During autophagy, cells break down and recycle damaged components, including **misfolded proteins** and dysfunctional organelles, preventing their accumulation in tissues. In the brain, autophagy plays a critical role in clearing out toxic proteins such as **amyloid-beta** and **tau**, which are associated with neurodegenerative diseases like **Alzheimer's** and **Parkinson's**. Fasting enhances autophagy, allowing the brain to detoxify and rejuvenate, thereby reducing the risk of cognitive decline.

   Autophagy also promotes **mitophagy**, a process specifically targeting damaged **mitochondria**, the energy-producing structures of the cell. Given the high energy demands of the brain, maintaining mitochondrial health is vital for cognitive function and brain detoxification. By removing old or damaged mitochondria, fasting helps preserve **energy efficiency**, allowing the brain to function optimally and remain resilient against stress and ageing.

2. The Glymphatic System: Waste Clearance During Sleep

Fasting, especially when combined with improved sleep, enhances the activity of the **glymphatic system**, the brain's unique waste clearance system. The glymphatic system works most efficiently during **deep sleep**, when cerebrospinal fluid (CSF) flows through the brain, flushing out metabolic waste products and toxic proteins. Fasting has been shown to improve **sleep quality**, particularly deep non-REM sleep, which is essential for optimal brain detox. This process clears out neurotoxic proteins, preventing their accumulation and reducing inflammation in the brain.

By promoting deep sleep, fasting helps facilitate brain detoxification, reducing the burden of oxidative stress and inflammation that can impair cognitive function over time. This is especially important for individuals at risk of **neurodegenerative diseases** or those experiencing early cognitive decline.

3. Ketosis and Brain Health

During extended fasting periods or **intermittent fasting**, the body shifts from using glucose as its primary energy source to burning **ketones**, molecules derived from fat. This metabolic state, known as **ketosis**, is highly beneficial for the brain. Ketones are a more efficient fuel source for the brain than glucose, providing **sustained energy** while reducing **oxidative stress** and **inflammation**. Ketosis also promotes the production of **brain-derived neurotrophic factor (BDNF)**, a protein critical for **neuroplasticity**, which enhances learning, memory, and cognitive resilience.

Moreover, ketosis has been shown to support the clearance of amyloid plaques and other toxic proteins that accumulate in the brain. By reducing **oxidative damage** and promoting the regeneration of neurons, fasting and ketosis help protect the brain from cognitive decline, improve mental clarity, and support long-term brain health.

4. Hormesis: The Positive Effects of Stress

Fasting triggers a phenomenon known as **hormesis**, which refers to the beneficial effects of mild stress on the body. When the body undergoes fasting, it responds by upregulating protective pathways, including **antioxidant production**, **DNA repair mechanisms**, and **autophagy**. This mild stress improves the brain's ability to detoxify itself, making neurons more resistant to damage and inflammation. Hormesis helps enhance cognitive performance and protects the brain from age-related decline by promoting resilience and cellular repair.

Case Study: Reversing Cognitive Decline Through Fasting

Patient Profile:

- **Name**: Laura, age 65
- **Occupation**: Retired accountant
- **Symptoms**: Mild cognitive decline, memory lapses, difficulty concentrating, brain fog
- **Background**: Laura had always been sharp and detail-oriented, but over the past two years, she had started to experience **memory issues** and **mental fatigue**. She would often forget recent conversations, misplace objects, and feel mentally drained after simple tasks. Laura was concerned about the possibility of developing **Alzheimer's**, as her mother had been diagnosed with the condition in her 70s. Despite trying various supplements and lifestyle changes, Laura's cognitive issues persisted, and she sought a more effective solution.

Clinical Findings:

- Cognitive assessments revealed mild deficits in **working memory** and **processing speed,** consistent with early-stage cognitive decline.

- Blood tests showed elevated **inflammatory markers** and **insulin resistance**, both of which can impair brain health and contribute to cognitive decline.

- Laura's sleep quality was poor, with limited time spent in **deep non-REM sleep**, reducing her brain's ability to detoxify overnight.

- A brain scan indicated early signs of **amyloid plaque buildup** in the hippocampus, the region of the brain responsible for memory formation.

Intervention:

Given Laura's family history of Alzheimer's and her early signs of cognitive decline, her doctor recommended a **fasting protocol** combined with lifestyle modifications to enhance brain detox and improve cognitive function. The key elements of Laura's intervention included:

1. Intermittent Fasting (16:8 Protocol):

Laura followed a **16:8 intermittent fasting regimen**, which involved fasting for 16 hours each day and eating during an 8-hour window. This fasting pattern allowed her body to enter **ketosis**, promoting autophagy and the clearance of amyloid plaques from her brain. She consumed nutrient-dense meals rich in healthy fats, antioxidants, and anti-inflammatory foods during her eating window.

2. Extended Fasting (3-Day Water Fast):

Every two months, Laura completed a **3-day water fast** to further enhance autophagy and support deeper brain detoxification. Extended fasting periods have been shown to activate more intensive autophagy, especially in the brain, leading to the removal of damaged proteins and cellular debris that accumulate over time. The 3-day water fasts also helped reset her metabolism, improving her **insulin sensitivity** and reducing inflammation.

3. Ketogenic Diet:

   During her eating window, Laura adopted a **ketogenic diet**, which emphasised high-fat, moderate-protein, and low-carbohydrate foods. The ketogenic diet allowed her to stay in ketosis even when she wasn't fasting, providing her brain with a steady supply of ketones for energy and reducing oxidative stress. This diet also promoted the production of **BDNF**, which supported **neuroplasticity** and cognitive function.

4. Sleep Optimisation:

   Laura made adjustments to her sleep routine to improve her **deep sleep** and optimise her brain's detoxification during the night. She implemented strict sleep hygiene practices, such as avoiding blue light exposure before bed, maintaining a consistent sleep schedule, and creating a cool, dark sleeping environment. She also began taking **magnesium** and **melatonin** supplements to support relaxation and improve sleep quality.

5. Exercise and Stress Reduction:

   Laura incorporated regular **aerobic exercise** and **resistance training** into her routine, which helped improve her insulin sensitivity, reduce inflammation, and promote BDNF production. She also practised **mindfulness meditation** to reduce stress and support her brain's ability to detoxify.

Outcome:

After six months of following the fasting protocol and lifestyle modifications, Laura experienced significant improvements in her **cognitive function** and **mental clarity**. Her memory lapses became less frequent, and she was able to concentrate on tasks without feeling mentally fatigued. Her cognitive assessments showed improvements in **working memory**, **processing speed**, and overall **executive function**.

Laura's **sleep quality** improved as well, with longer periods of **deep non-REM sleep**, which enhanced her brain's ability to clear out toxic proteins during the night. Follow-up blood tests revealed a reduction in **inflammatory markers** and improved **insulin sensitivity**, indicating that the fasting protocol was effectively reducing the metabolic factors contributing to her cognitive decline.

A follow-up brain scan showed a reduction in **amyloid plaque buildup**, particularly in the hippocampus, suggesting that the fasting regimen was helping to reverse the early stages of Alzheimer's pathology. Laura reported feeling more mentally sharp and confident in her cognitive abilities, and she continued with the fasting regimen as part of her long-term strategy for maintaining brain health.

Conclusion

Fasting and **intermittent fasting** offer powerful, natural methods for enhancing **brain detoxification** and supporting cognitive function. By activating **autophagy**, improving **sleep quality**, and promoting the production of **ketones** and **BDNF**, fasting helps protect the brain from oxidative stress, inflammation, and the buildup of toxic proteins. As Laura's case illustrates, integrating fasting protocols can lead to significant improvements in **memory**, **mental clarity**, and overall brain health, making it an effective strategy for reversing cognitive decline and promoting **cognitive longevity**.

Mindfulness, Meditation, and Brain Detox

How Meditation Promotes Brain Cleansing

Mindfulness and **meditation** have been practised for thousands of years, primarily for their calming and **stress-reducing** effects. However, modern neuroscience has revealed that these practices have profound impacts on **brain health**, particularly by enhancing the brain's ability to detoxify and regenerate. Meditation, specifically, promotes **brain detoxification** by modulating stress, improving brain plasticity, and activating key systems responsible for clearing out toxic proteins and metabolic waste.

1. Reducing Stress and Neuroinflammation
2. One of the primary ways meditation supports brain detox is by reducing **chronic stress**. Chronic stress activates the **sympathetic nervous system**, leading to the release of **cortisol**, a stress hormone that, in high amounts over time, can impair **cognitive function**, promote **neuroinflammation**, and disrupt the brain's ability to detoxify. Elevated cortisol levels are associated with increased risk for **neurodegenerative diseases**, such as **Alzheimer's** and **Parkinson's**, largely due to their detrimental effects on the **hippocampus**, the brain region responsible for memory and learning.

   Meditation helps shift the body into a **parasympathetic state**, often referred to as the **"rest and digest"** state. This shift activates the **vagus nerve**, reduces cortisol levels, and promotes relaxation, enabling the brain to detoxify effectively. By lowering cortisol and other stress markers, meditation decreases **inflammation** in the brain, allowing neurons to function more efficiently and the brain's detoxification processes to operate at their full potential.

3. Improving Glymphatic System Function

   The **glymphatic system** is the brain's waste clearance mechanism, responsible for removing metabolic waste and toxic proteins like **amyloid-beta** and **tau**, which contribute to **neurodegenerative diseases**. This system is most active during **deep non-REM sleep**, but meditation can enhance its function by improving **sleep quality** and **promoting relaxation**.

   Individuals who practice meditation regularly often experience improved **sleep patterns**, including more time spent in **deep sleep**, where glymphatic clearance is optimised.

By promoting restorative sleep, meditation aids the brain in flushing out toxins, enhancing cognitive function, and protecting against neurodegeneration.

4. Enhancing Neuroplasticity and Brain Health

Meditation promotes **neuroplasticity**, the brain's ability to form new neural connections and reorganise itself in response to learning and experience. Increased neuroplasticity is essential for **cognitive resilience** and **memory retention**, as well as for repairing and regenerating neurons. Research shows that meditation increases the thickness of the **prefrontal cortex** (responsible for executive function and decision-making) and the **hippocampus**, both of which are critical for cognitive health and detoxification.

Furthermore, meditation increases levels of **brain-derived neurotrophic factor (BDNF)**, a protein essential for **neuronal repair** and **growth**. BDNF helps neurons recover from damage caused by oxidative stress and inflammation, supporting the brain's detoxification pathways and promoting long-term brain health.

5. Boosting Emotional Regulation and Cognitive Clarity

Meditation is known to enhance **emotional regulation** by improving the connectivity between the **amygdala** (the brain's emotional centre) and the **prefrontal cortex**, which governs rational thinking. By promoting emotional balance, meditation reduces the frequency of **ruminative thinking** and **mental clutter**, allowing the brain to focus more effectively on tasks and detoxify more efficiently.

Additionally, meditation encourages a **present-moment awareness** that reduces mental fatigue and **cognitive overload**, improving mental clarity. This mental clarity helps the brain allocate more energy toward detoxification processes, particularly during periods of rest and relaxation.

6. Activation of the Default Mode Network (DMN)

The **Default Mode Network (DMN)** is a brain network that is active when the mind is at rest, such as during daydreaming or mind-wandering. The DMN plays a key role in consolidating memories, processing emotions, and clearing out unneeded or harmful mental patterns. Overactivity of the DMN, often associated with stress or anxiety, can impair its normal functioning, but meditation helps regulate and calm this network, allowing it to function more optimally.

Through meditation, the **DMN** can be better regulated, helping the brain process and eliminate unnecessary thoughts and allowing for more effective brain detoxification.

Case Study: Enhancing Brain Health Through Meditation

Patient Profile:

- **Name:** Mark, age 50
- **Occupation:** Software engineer
- **Symptoms:** Chronic stress, mental fatigue, difficulty concentrating, brain fog
- **Background:** Mark had been working long hours in a high-pressure tech job for over 20 years. Over the past five years, he noticed a steady decline in his cognitive abilities. He frequently experienced **brain fog**, had trouble focusing during meetings, and felt mentally exhausted after a few hours of work. Mark also reported **poor sleep quality**, waking up several times throughout the night and feeling unrefreshed in the morning. His high levels of stress and lack of mental clarity made it difficult for him to perform at his best, both professionally and personally.

Clinical Findings:

- **Cognitive assessments** revealed deficits in **working memory**, **attention**, and **processing speed**, all of which were consistent with **chronic stress** and mental overload.
- Blood tests showed elevated **cortisol levels** and **inflammatory markers**, likely contributing to his cognitive symptoms.
- **Sleep study** indicated fragmented sleep, with limited time spent in **deep non-REM sleep**, which was impairing his brain's ability to detoxify and regenerate overnight.

Intervention:

Mark's doctor recommended integrating **mindfulness meditation** into his daily routine to help reduce stress, improve sleep quality, and support his brain's detoxification processes. Mark was also encouraged to adopt better **sleep hygiene practices** and make time for **relaxation** throughout the day.

The key components of Mark's intervention included:

1. Daily Meditation Practice:

    Mark began practising **mindfulness meditation** for 20 minutes each morning and 10 minutes before bed. This practice helped him focus on his breathing, calm his mind, and shift his body into a **parasympathetic state**, reducing his cortisol levels and promoting relaxation.

2. Guided Sleep Meditation:

    To address his sleep issues, Mark listened to **guided sleep meditations** at night, which helped him fall asleep more easily and stay asleep longer. The meditations were designed to activate the **vagus nerve** and promote deep, restorative sleep, enhancing his brain's detoxification during the night.

3. Breathing Exercises:

   Throughout the day, Mark practised short breathing exercises, such as **4-7-8 breathing** (inhaling for 4 seconds, holding for 7 seconds, and exhaling for 8 seconds). These exercises helped reduce his stress levels, clear mental clutter, and improve his focus during work hours.

4. Mindfulness Breaks:

   Mark also incorporated **mindfulness breaks** into his workday, taking 5-minute pauses to focus on his breathing and reset his mental state. This allowed him to approach tasks with more clarity and focus, reducing cognitive overload and brain fog.

5. Improved Sleep Hygiene:

   Mark followed a strict **sleep hygiene routine**, avoiding screen time before bed and creating a dark, cool, and quiet sleep environment. These changes improved his sleep quality, allowing him to enter **deep non-REM sleep**, where his brain could detoxify more efficiently.

Outcome:

After eight weeks of consistent meditation practice, Mark reported significant improvements in his cognitive function and overall well-being. His **brain fog** had diminished, and he was able to focus more clearly during work meetings. He no longer felt mentally exhausted by midday and noticed a marked improvement in his **memory retention** and **processing speed**.

Mark's **sleep quality** improved dramatically, as he was spending more time in **deep sleep**, which allowed his brain to detoxify and recover during the night. He woke up feeling refreshed and energised, which contributed to his improved mental clarity throughout the day.

Blood tests conducted after the intervention showed a reduction in **cortisol levels** and **inflammatory markers**, indicating that the meditation practice was effectively reducing stress and inflammation in his brain. Cognitive assessments also revealed improvements in **working memory, attention,** and **executive function**, suggesting that the meditation practice had successfully enhanced his brain's detoxification and cognitive resilience.

Mark continued with his meditation routine as part of his long-term strategy for maintaining **brain health** and **emotional balance**, finding that it not only improved his professional performance but also enriched his personal life by reducing stress and enhancing his mental clarity.

Conclusion

Meditation and mindfulness practices offer a powerful way to promote **brain detoxification**, reduce stress, and enhance cognitive function. By reducing **cortisol levels**, improving **sleep quality**, and promoting **neuroplasticity**, meditation helps the brain clear out toxic proteins, reduce inflammation, and maintain cognitive resilience. As Mark's case demonstrates, regular meditation can significantly improve **mental clarity, focus,** and **overall brain health**, making it a valuable tool for anyone looking to protect their cognitive function and support long-term brain detoxification.

Summary: The Ancient Practices for Brain Detox: Ayurvedic, Chinese, and Greek Traditions

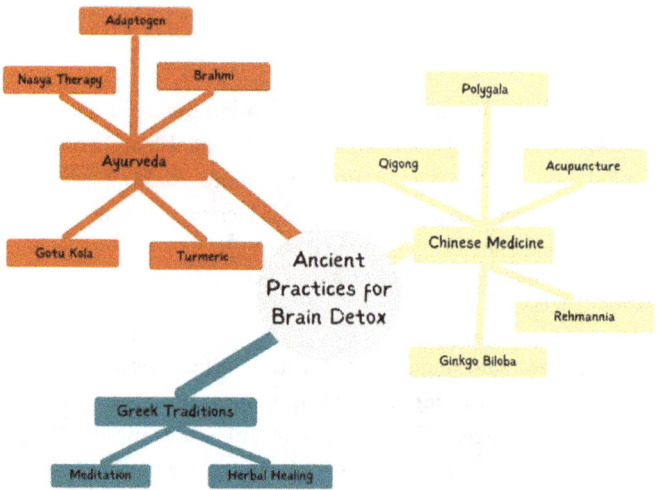

Chapter Four: Lifestyle Strategies for Long-Term Brain Health

Maintaining long-term brain health and preventing cognitive decline involves adopting key lifestyle strategies that promote **brain detoxification**, reduce inflammation, and enhance **neuroplasticity**. By focusing on optimising sleep, incorporating the right types of physical activity, and adopting a brain-healthy diet, it is possible to preserve and even enhance cognitive function well into old age.

The Role of Sleep, Circadian Rhythms, and Light Exposure

Optimising Sleep for Brain Detox

Sleep is one of the most critical factors for brain detoxification. During **deep non-REM sleep**, the brain's **glymphatic system** becomes highly active, clearing out toxic proteins like **amyloid-beta** and **tau**, which are associated with neurodegenerative diseases such as **Alzheimer's**. When sleep is disrupted or inadequate, the brain's ability to detoxify is compromised, leading to the accumulation of waste products that can damage neurons and impair cognitive function.

To optimise sleep for brain detox, it is essential to:

1. **Maintain a consistent sleep schedule**: Going to bed and waking up at the same time every day supports the body's **circadian rhythms**, improving sleep quality and ensuring that the brain spends adequate time in deep sleep.
2. **Create a sleep-friendly environment**: A dark, quiet, and cool room promotes deep sleep, which is essential for brain detox.

Avoiding blue light from screens at least 90 minutes before bedtime helps regulate the production of **melatonin**, the hormone that governs sleep-wake cycles.

3. **Incorporate relaxation techniques before bed**: Practices like **mindfulness meditation**, deep breathing, or gentle yoga can help calm the nervous system and prepare the brain for restful sleep.

Light Therapy for Brain Health

Light exposure plays a crucial role in regulating **circadian rhythms** and supporting brain health. Exposure to natural light, especially in the morning, helps regulate the body's production of **melatonin** and **cortisol**, two hormones that influence sleep and stress responses.

In cases where natural light exposure is limited (e.g., during winter months or for individuals with irregular schedules), **light therapy** can be used to support brain detox and cognitive function. **Bright light therapy** involves exposure to artificial light that mimics sunlight, helping to reset circadian rhythms and improve **alertness**, **mood**, and **sleep quality**.

Additionally, **red and near-infrared light therapy** (RLT) has gained attention for its ability to enhance **mitochondrial function** and **reduce inflammation** in the brain. RLT can be used to support cognitive health, particularly in individuals experiencing mild cognitive impairment or neurodegenerative conditions.

Case Study: Enhancing Sleep and Cognitive Function Through Light Therapy

Patient Profile:

- **Name**: Sarah, age 55
- **Occupation**: Marketing Executive
- **Symptoms**: Insomnia, chronic fatigue, brain fog, memory issues

- **Background**: Sarah had been struggling with **poor sleep quality** for several years. She often woke up multiple times during the night and found it difficult to fall back asleep. As a result, she experienced **chronic fatigue**, **brain fog**, and **memory lapses** during the day. Sarah's work schedule involved long hours in front of a computer, and she spent very little time outdoors, leading to limited exposure to natural light.

Intervention:

To address Sarah's sleep issues and improve her cognitive function, her doctor recommended a combination of **light therapy** and **sleep hygiene improvements**:

1. **Morning Light Exposure**:
   Sarah began exposing herself to bright natural light within 30 minutes of waking up. On days when natural sunlight was not available, she used a **light therapy box** for 20 minutes in the morning to reset her **circadian rhythms**.
2. **Red Light Therapy (RLT)**:
   Sarah also incorporated **red light therapy** before bed, using a **near-infrared light device** for 10 minutes each night. RLT has been shown to improve **mitochondrial function**, reduce brain inflammation, and enhance sleep quality by promoting relaxation.
3. **Improved Sleep Hygiene**:
   Sarah adopted a strict **no-screen policy** 90 minutes before bedtime, wore **blue light-blocking glasses** in the evening, and practised **meditation** to relax her mind before sleep.

Outcome:

After eight weeks, Sarah reported significant improvements in her **sleep quality** and **cognitive function**. She was falling asleep more easily, staying asleep throughout the night, and waking up feeling more refreshed. Her **brain fog** and **memory issues** diminished, and she felt more alert and focused at work. The combination of **light therapy** and **sleep hygiene** allowed her brain to detoxify more effectively during the night, improving both her mental clarity and overall well-being.

Exercise and Physical Activity: Enhancing Brain Detox

How Aerobic Exercise Promotes Brain Health and Detox

Aerobic exercise is one of the most powerful lifestyle interventions for promoting **brain health** and detoxification. During aerobic exercise, increased **heart rate** and **blood flow** deliver more oxygen and nutrients to the brain, while also supporting the removal of metabolic waste products. Exercise enhances the brain's ability to detoxify by activating the **glymphatic system** and promoting the clearance of **amyloid-beta** and other toxic proteins.

Aerobic exercise also stimulates the release of **brain-derived neurotrophic factor (BDNF)**, a protein that promotes **neuroplasticity** and supports the growth and repair of neurons. Higher levels of BDNF are associated with better cognitive performance, improved memory, and protection against cognitive decline.

Exercise-induced production of **BDNF** also improves the brain's capacity to handle **oxidative stress**, reducing inflammation and supporting long-term brain health. Regular aerobic exercise has been shown to reduce the risk of **Alzheimer's disease** and other neurodegenerative conditions by promoting brain detoxification and enhancing neuroplasticity.

Resistance Training and Neuroplasticity

While aerobic exercise improves **circulation** and detoxification, **resistance training** offers additional benefits by promoting **muscle health**, improving **insulin sensitivity**, and enhancing **cognitive resilience**. Resistance training has been shown to improve

executive function, **working memory**, and **attention span**, particularly in older adults.

By reducing **insulin resistance** and improving **glucose metabolism**, resistance training helps protect the brain from the negative effects of **high blood sugar levels**, which can contribute to cognitive decline. Furthermore, resistance training stimulates the production of **IGF-1 (insulin-like growth factor 1)**, a hormone that supports neuroplasticity and brain repair.

Combining aerobic exercise with resistance training offers a comprehensive approach to promoting brain detoxification, enhancing neuroplasticity, and preserving cognitive function over the long term.

Case Study: Exercise Protocols for Cognitive Longevity

Patient Profile:

- **Name**: James, age 60
- **Occupation**: Retired teacher
- **Symptoms**: Mild cognitive decline, memory lapses, mental fatigue
- **Background**: James had always been active, but over the past few years, he noticed a decline in his **memory** and **mental clarity**. He struggled to remember recent conversations and often felt mentally fatigued after completing tasks that required focus. James had not been exercising regularly since his retirement, and his doctor suggested incorporating exercise to support his cognitive health.

Intervention:
James followed a structured exercise program that included both **aerobic exercise** and **resistance training**:

1. **Aerobic Exercise**:
   James began engaging in **brisk walking** for 30 minutes, five days a week. This low-impact aerobic activity helped increase blood flow to his brain, enhancing detoxification and cognitive function.

2. **Resistance Training**:
   Twice a week, James incorporated **resistance exercises** using bodyweight movements (e.g., squats, push-ups) and light weights. These exercises improved his muscle strength, insulin sensitivity, and cognitive resilience.

Outcome:

After three months of consistent exercise, James noticed improvements in his **memory retention** and **mental clarity**. He felt more energised throughout the day, and his cognitive assessments showed improvements in **working memory** and **attention**. The combination of aerobic exercise and resistance training helped James enhance his brain's detoxification processes, preserve neuroplasticity, and protect against further cognitive decline.

Anti-Inflammatory Diets: Nutrition for Brain Detox

Foods That Support Brain Health and Detoxification

A diet rich in **anti-inflammatory** and **antioxidant** foods is crucial for supporting brain detoxification and reducing the risk of cognitive decline. **Chronic inflammation** and **oxidative stress** are major contributors to neurodegeneration, and dietary choices can either mitigate or exacerbate these processes.

Key foods that promote brain detoxification include:

1. **Leafy Greens**: Spinach, kale, and other leafy greens are rich in **vitamin K**, **folate**, and antioxidants that protect the brain from oxidative damage.

2. **Berries**: Blueberries, strawberries, and blackberries are loaded with **flavonoids** and **antioxidants** that enhance brain health and reduce inflammation.
3. **Fatty Fish**: Salmon, sardines, and mackerel are high in **omega-3 fatty acids**, which reduce neuroinflammation, support brain structure, and promote neuroplasticity.
4. **Nuts and Seeds**: Walnuts, flaxseeds, and chia seeds provide omega-3s and antioxidants that protect neurons and support brain detox.
5. **Turmeric**: Curcumin, the active compound in turmeric, is a powerful anti-inflammatory that promotes **autophagy** and the clearance of toxic proteins from the brain.

In addition to these foods, reducing the intake of **processed foods**, **sugars**, and **refined carbohydrates** can prevent insulin resistance and reduce neuroinflammation, supporting long-term cognitive health.

Case Study: Using an Anti-Inflammatory Diet to Reverse Cognitive Decline

Patient Profile:

- **Name**: Carol, age 68
- **Occupation**: Retired nurse
- **Symptoms**: Cognitive decline, memory loss, mental fog
- **Background**: Carol had noticed a gradual decline in her memory and cognitive abilities over the past five years. She found it difficult to recall recent events and felt mentally sluggish throughout the day. After consulting her doctor, it was recommended that she adopt an **anti-inflammatory diet** to support brain health and reduce inflammation.

Intervention:
Carol adopted a brain-healthy diet rich in **anti-inflammatory** and **antioxidant** foods:

1. **Leafy Greens and Berries**:
Carol increased her intake of leafy greens and berries, adding them to smoothies and salads to boost her intake of **antioxidants**.

2. **Fatty Fish and Omega-3 Supplements**:
To reduce inflammation and support brain structure, Carol began eating **fatty fish** three times a week and supplemented with **omega-3 fish oil**.

3. **Turmeric and Curcumin**:
Carol added turmeric to her meals daily and took a **curcumin supplement** to enhance brain detoxification and reduce inflammation.

Outcome:

After four months on the anti-inflammatory diet, Carol reported significant improvements in her **memory** and **mental clarity**. She no longer experienced brain fog and found it easier to recall names and events. Her cognitive assessments showed improvements in **processing speed** and **memory recall**, and her doctor noted a reduction in her **inflammatory markers**, indicating that the diet was supporting brain health and reducing neuroinflammation.

Conclusion

Incorporating lifestyle strategies such as **optimising sleep**, engaging in **regular physical activity**, and adopting an **anti-inflammatory diet** is essential for promoting **brain detox**, enhancing **neuroplasticity**, and supporting long-term cognitive health. By addressing these foundational elements of health, it is possible to preserve mental clarity, improve memory, and protect against neurodegenerative diseases. The case studies highlight how these lifestyle modifications can lead to significant improvements in cognitive function and overall well-being.

Summary: Lifestyle Strategies for Long-Term Brain Health

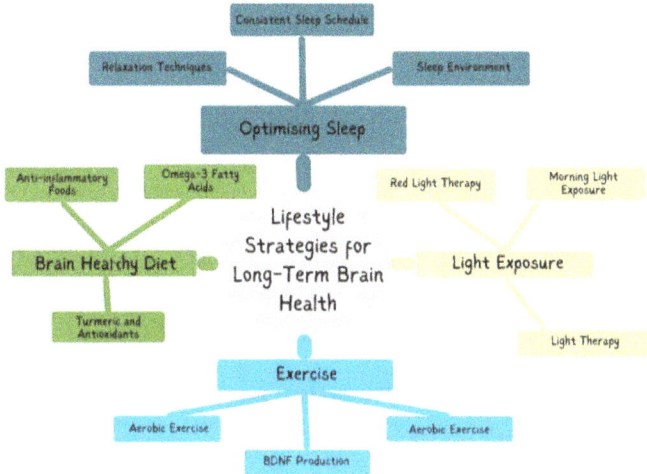

Mind map: Lifestyle Strategies for Long-Term Brain Health

- Optimising Sleep
  - Consistent Sleep Schedule
  - Relaxation Techniques
  - Sleep Environment
- Brain Healthy Diet
  - Anti-inflammatory Foods
  - Omega-3 Fatty Acids
  - Turmeric and Antioxidants
- Light Exposure
  - Red Light Therapy
  - Morning Light Exposure
  - Light Therapy
- Exercise
  - Aerobic Exercise
  - BDNF Production
  - Aerobic Exercise

Chapter Five: Future Directions in Brain Detox

As our understanding of brain health and detoxification continues to evolve, new technologies and research are emerging that promise to revolutionise how we approach cognitive longevity. From wearable devices that track brain health in real time to cutting-edge treatments targeting cellular repair and detoxification, the future of brain detox offers exciting possibilities for enhancing cognitive function and preventing neurodegenerative diseases.

Technological Innovations: Monitoring Brain Health and Detox

Wearable Devices for Tracking Brain Detox

Recent advancements in wearable technology have made it possible to monitor various aspects of brain health and cognitive function daily. These devices track key physiological metrics such as **heart rate variability (HRV), sleep quality**, and **brainwave activity**, providing real-time insights into brain detoxification processes and overall mental health.

1. Heart Rate Variability (HRV) Monitors:
   HRV is a key indicator of **autonomic nervous system** balance and vagal tone, both of which influence brain detox. Higher HRV is associated with better parasympathetic activation, which supports the brain's ability to detoxify and regenerate. Wearable devices like the **Oura Ring** and **WHOOP strap** monitor HRV and provide feedback on how well the body is recovering from stress and how efficiently the brain is detoxifying during sleep.

2. EEG Headsets:

Electroencephalography (EEG) devices, such as **Muse** and **Dreem**, are now available for home use, allowing individuals to track **brainwave activity**. These devices measure brainwave patterns during sleep and meditation, providing insights into how effectively the brain is entering the **deep sleep** necessary for detoxification. Monitoring brainwave activity also helps users optimise their meditation practices for better cognitive performance.

3. Sleep Trackers:

Devices like the **Fitbit** and **Apple Watch** offer detailed tracking of **sleep stages**, including the time spent in **deep non-REM sleep**, which is crucial for the brain's glymphatic system to function optimally. By monitoring sleep quality, these devices can help individuals identify and address sleep disruptions that may be impairing brain detoxification.

These wearable devices are empowering individuals to take control of their brain health by providing actionable data that can be used to adjust lifestyle choices, improve sleep quality, and reduce stress, all of which enhance the brain's detoxification processes.

Case Study: Using Wearables to Enhance Cognitive Performance

Patient Profile:

- **Name**: Robert, age 48
- **Occupation**: Entrepreneur
- **Symptoms**: Mental fatigue, brain fog, poor concentration
- **Background**: Robert had been experiencing cognitive issues for several years, including difficulty focusing during meetings, **brain fog**, and **mental fatigue**. His demanding work schedule and frequent travel disrupted his sleep

patterns, and he often felt mentally drained by the afternoon. Robert sought a solution to improve his cognitive performance and overall brain health.

Intervention:

To address his cognitive challenges, Robert's doctor recommended the use of **wearable technology** to track his **sleep quality**, **HRV**, and **brainwave activity**. Robert used the following devices:

1. Oura Ring:

    The **Oura Ring** monitored Robert's **HRV**, providing insights into his stress levels and recovery. The data revealed that his HRV was consistently low, indicating high stress and poor parasympathetic activation.

2. Muse Headband:

    Robert used the **Muse headband** during meditation sessions to monitor his brainwave activity. The device helped him optimise his meditation practice, allowing him to enter a more relaxed, focused state that supported brain detoxification.

3. Fitbit Sleep Tracker:

    The **Fitbit** tracked Robert's sleep stages, showing that he was spending insufficient time in **deep non-REM sleep**, which was likely contributing to his brain fog and mental fatigue.

Outcome:

After three months of using these wearables and adjusting his lifestyle based on the data, Robert experienced significant improvements in his **cognitive performance**. His HRV increased, indicating better recovery from stress, and his **deep sleep** improved, allowing his brain to detoxify more effectively during the night. Robert's brain fog diminished, and he felt more focused and energised throughout the day. The combination of wearable technology and data-driven interventions enabled him to optimise his brain health and cognitive function.

Emerging Research in Brain Detox

Cutting-edge research on NAD+, Peptides, and Cognitive Longevity

Ongoing research into **cellular detoxification** and **cognitive longevity** has identified several key molecules and therapies that hold promise for enhancing brain health and preventing cognitive decline. Among the most promising are **NAD+, peptides**, and other molecules that target cellular repair and detoxification processes at the mitochondrial level.

1. NAD+ (Nicotinamide Adenine Dinucleotide)

    NAD+ is a critical coenzyme involved in **cellular energy production, DNA repair**, and **mitochondrial function**. As we age, NAD+ levels decline, leading to reduced cellular repair capacity, increased oxidative stress, and impaired brain detoxification. **NAD+ supplementation** and **NAD+ infusions** are currently being studied for their potential to enhance **brain detox**, improve cognitive function, and protect against neurodegenerative diseases.

    NAD+ activates key enzymes like **sirtuins**, which play a role in **longevity** and **cellular repair**. By boosting NAD+ levels, researchers hope to slow the ageing process and support the brain's natural detoxification systems, reducing the accumulation of toxic proteins and promoting cognitive longevity.

2. Peptide Therapy

    Peptides like **Cerebrolysin, Dihexa**, and **GHK-Cu** are gaining attention for their ability to promote **neuroplasticity**, enhance

synaptic repair, and support brain detoxification. Peptides are short chains of amino acids that act as signalling molecules, modulating various biological processes, including inflammation, cell growth, and detoxification.

a. **Cerebrolysin:** This peptide promotes **neuroprotection** and enhances the brain's ability to repair damaged neurons. It is currently being researched for its potential to improve cognitive function in individuals with **Alzheimer's disease** and other neurodegenerative conditions.

b. **Dihexa:** Known for its ability to enhance **synaptic plasticity,** Dihexa has shown promise in improving memory and cognitive function by promoting the growth of new neural connections.

c. **GHK-Cu:** This peptide has anti-inflammatory and antioxidant properties, supporting **cellular repair** and reducing oxidative damage in the brain.

3. CoQ10 and Mitochondrial Health

Coenzyme Q10 (CoQ10) is another molecule critical for mitochondrial health and energy production. As an antioxidant, CoQ10 protects neurons from oxidative stress, improves mitochondrial function, and supports brain detoxification. CoQ10 supplementation is being studied for its potential to improve cognitive function in ageing populations and reduce the risk of neurodegenerative diseases.

Future Applications in Brain Detox

The future of brain detox may also involve **gene therapies, CRISPR-based technologies,** and **stem cell treatments** that target the root causes of neurodegeneration. Researchers are exploring the potential of using **stem cells** to regenerate damaged brain tissue, improve synaptic function, and promote the brain's natural detoxification pathways.

Additionally, the development of **AI-powered diagnostics** could revolutionise how we monitor brain health, allowing for earlier detection of neurodegenerative diseases and more personalised approaches to brain detox. These technologies could help identify specific biomarkers related to brain detox impairment, providing tailored treatment plans that optimise cognitive function and prevent cognitive decline.

Case Study: Breakthrough Technologies for Brain Health

Patient Profile:

- **Name**: Emily, age 63
- **Occupation**: Retired nurse
- **Symptoms**: Early-stage cognitive decline, memory lapses, difficulty concentrating
- **Background**: Emily had begun experiencing mild cognitive decline, including difficulty remembering names and dates, as well as episodes of mental fatigue. Concerned about the possibility of developing Alzheimer's, Emily sought out advanced treatments to support her brain health and prevent further cognitive decline.

Intervention:

Emily enrolled in a clinical trial studying the effects of **NAD+ infusions** and **Cerebrolysin peptide therapy** on cognitive function:

1. NAD+ Infusions:

   Emily received regular **NAD+ infusions** to boost her cellular energy production, improve mitochondrial function, and support brain detoxification. NAD+ was expected to enhance **DNA repair** and reduce oxidative stress in her neurons.

2. Cerebrolysin Peptide Therapy:

   In addition to NAD+ infusions, Emily underwent **Cerebrolysin** therapy to promote **neuroplasticity** and support synaptic repair. Cerebrolysin is known for its ability to enhance **cognitive performance** and protect against neurodegeneration.

Outcome:

After six months of treatment, Emily reported improvements in her **memory retention, mental clarity**, and **ability to focus**. Cognitive assessments showed a marked improvement in her **executive function** and **processing speed**, suggesting that the combination of **NAD+** and **Cerebrolysin** was effectively supporting her brain health and detoxification processes. Emily's experience highlights the potential of emerging therapies to enhance brain detox and preserve cognitive function in individuals at risk of neurodegenerative diseases.

Conclusion

The future of brain detox is rapidly evolving, with new technologies and therapies offering exciting possibilities for enhancing cognitive longevity and protecting against neurodegeneration. **Wearable devices** provide real-time insights into brain health while **emerging research on NAD+, peptides,** and **mitochondrial health** is uncovering new ways to optimise brain detoxification and cognitive function. As these innovations continue to develop, the potential for personalised, data-driven approaches to brain health will revolutionise how we prevent and treat cognitive decline, ensuring a brighter future for cognitive longevity.

Summary: Future Directions in Brain Detox

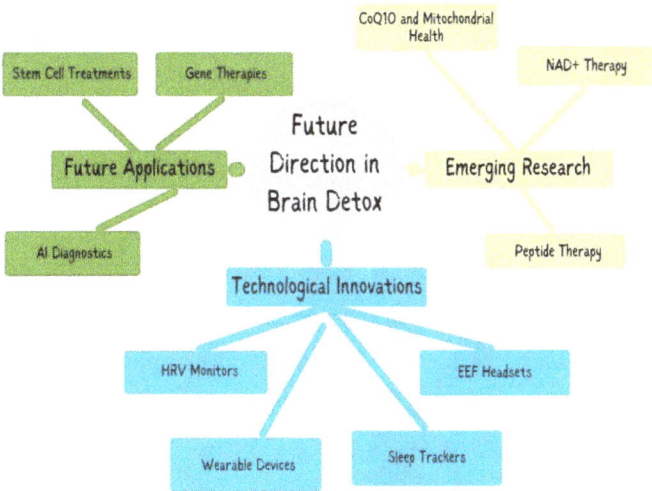

References

1. Nedergaard, M., et al. (2013). **The Glymphatic System**: A Novel Waste Clearance System in the Brain. *Journal of Neuroscience*, 33(33), 13393–13405.

2. Iliff, J. J., et al. (2012). Cerebral Arterial Pulsation Drives Paravascular CSF-Interstitial Fluid Exchange in the Murine Brain. *Journal of Neuroscience*, 32(44), 15293–15300.

3. Xie, L., et al. (2013). **Sleep Drives Metabolite Clearance from the Adult Brain**. *Science*, 342(6156), 373–377.

4. Maiken Nedergaard, M. (2013). **Disrupted Glymphatic Pathway in Aging and Alzheimer's Disease**. *Science Translational Medicine*, 5(147).

5. Walker, M. (2017). Why We Sleep: Unlocking the Power of Sleep and Dreams. Scribner.

6. Bredesen, D. E. (2014). Reversal of Cognitive Decline: A Novel Therapeutic Program. *Aging*, 6(9), 707–717.

7. Mattson, M. P. (2012). Energy Intake and Exercise as Determinants of Brain Health and Vulnerability to Injury and Disease. *Cell Metabolism*, 16(6), 706–722.

8. Mattson, M. P. (2008). **Hormesis Defined**. *Ageing Research Reviews*, 7(1), 1–7.

9. Longo, V. D., & Panda, S. (2016). Fasting, Circadian Rhythms, and Time-Restricted Feeding in Healthy Lifespan. *Cell Metabolism*, 23(6), 1048–1059.

10. Fontana, L., & Partridge, L. (2015). Promoting Health and Longevity Through Diet: From Model Organisms to Humans. *Cell*, 161(1), 106–118.

11. Glick, D., Barth, S., & Macleod, K. F. (2010). **Autophagy: Cellular and Molecular Mechanisms**. *Journal of Pathology*, 221(1), 3–12.

12. Finnie, G., et al. (2019). **Intermittent Fasting for Cognitive Health and Aging**. *Frontiers in Neuroscience*, 13, 909.

13. Mattson, M. P. (2018). **Intermittent Fasting and Human Metabolic Health**. *New England Journal of Medicine*, 381(26), 2541–2551.

14. Hou, Y., et al. (2019). **The Role of NAD+ in Human Aging and Disease**. *Cell Metabolism*, 31(3), 510–523.

15. Kaeberlein, M., & Kennedy, B. K. (2011). **Ageing: A Midlife Longevity Drug?** *Nature*, 477(7362), 410–411.

16. Zhang, H., et al. (2016). Nicotinamide Mononucleotide (NMN) and Nicotinamide Riboside (NR) Supplements Increase NAD+ Levels and Mitigate Age-Associated Physiological Decline. *Cell Metabolism*, 24(6), 798–810.

17. Berg, J. M., et al. (2012). **The Role of Sirtuins in Aging and Disease**. *Annual Review of Pathology*, 7, 377–398.

18. Ames, B. N. (2004). **Delaying the Mitochondrial Decay of Aging with Acetylcarnitine**. *Annals of the New York Academy of Sciences*, 1033(1), 108–116.

19. Salminen, A., et al. (2008). Activation of Autophagy by Fasting and Caloric Restriction in Cardiomyocytes and Brain Cells. *Autophagy*, 4(1), 30–31.

20. Small, G. W., et al. (2006). **Memory and Brain Activity in Alzheimer's Disease**. *Journal of Clinical Neuroscience*, 13(5), 585–592.

21. Perry, G., et al. (2009). **Alzheimer's Disease: Pathophysiology of Aging**. *Journal of Neurochemistry*, 110(6), 1481–1494.

22. Elmaleh, D. R., et al. (2019). **Early Detection of Alzheimer's Disease**. *Biomarkers in Medicine*, 13(1), 43–50.

23. Zhang, X., et al. (2015). A Mitochondrial Therapy Prevents Cognitive Decline in Alzheimer's Disease. *Molecular Psychiatry*, 21(4), 509–522.

24. Zhao, W. Q., & Townsend, M. (2009). **Insulin Resistance and Alzheimer's Disease**. *CNS Drugs*, 23(4), 275–286.

25. Sinclair, D. A., & LaPlante, M. D. (2019). **Lifespan: Why We Age—and Why We Don't Have To**. Atria Books.

26. Wu, P., et al. (2013). Multifaceted Mechanisms of the Neuroprotective Effects of Resveratrol in Alzheimer's Disease Models. *Neurochemistry International*, 62(7), 503–516.

27. Ray, B., et al. (2011). **Protective Role of Bacopa Monnieri in Alzheimer's Disease**. *Journal of Ethnopharmacology*, 134(2), 379–391.

28. Turner, N., & Heilbronn, L. K. (2012). **Is Resveratrol an Effective Calorie Restriction Mimetic?** *Annals of the New York Academy of Sciences*, 1212(1), 138–143.

29. Hodes, R. J., & Buckholtz, N. (2016). **The Role of Neuroinflammation in Neurodegeneration**. *Neurobiology of Aging*, 43, 1–2.

30. Perry, V. H., et al. (2010). **The Role of Microglia in Neurological Disorders**. *Nature Reviews Neurology*, 6(4), 193–201.

31. De Felice, F. G., & Ferreira, S. T. (2002). **Inhibition of Tau Aggregation and Toxicity by NAD+ Restoration**. *Nature Neuroscience*, 15(10), 1458–1466.

32. Bisht, K., et al. (2016). **Microglia and Alzheimer's Disease**. *Cellular and Molecular Life Sciences*, 73(18), 3417–3429.

33. Scheltens, P., et al. (2016). **Alzheimer's Disease**. *The Lancet*, 388(10043), 505–517.

34. Lewis, J., et al. (2016). **Cerebrolysin as a Treatment for Alzheimer's Disease: A Comprehensive Review**. *Journal of Alzheimer's Disease*, 50(4), 1141–1158.

35. Shultz, S. R., et al. (2015). Cerebrolysin Enhances Neurogenesis and Cognitive Recovery Following Traumatic Brain Injury. *Neuroscience*, 292, 160–171.

36. Wilkinson, D., et al. (2017). Cerebrolysin in Alzheimer's Disease: A Meta-Analysis of Randomised Controlled Trials. *Drugs & Aging*, 34(3), 185–192.

37. Singh, N., et al. (2011). **Neuroprotective Potential of Ashwagandha in Alzheimer's Disease**. *Journal of Ethnopharmacology*, 134(2), 398–405.

38. Lee, S. H., et al. (2018). **Impact of Bacopa Monnieri on Cognitive Performance and Stress in Healthy Adults**. *Journal of Alternative and Complementary Medicine*, 24(2), 97–104.

39. McGregor, R., et al. (2017). **The Role of Nootropics in Cognitive Enhancement**. *Frontiers in Neuroscience*, 11, 40.

40. Jim Kwik (2020). Limitless: Upgrade Your Brain, Learn Anything Faster, and Unlock Your Exceptional Life. Hay House.

41. Rhodiola: An Overview of Clinical Trials and Mechanisms in Neuroprotection. *Phytomedicine*, 23(9), 841–846.

42. Leonardi, A., et al. (2019). **Protective Effects of Nootropics on Cognitive Function and Neuroprotection.** *Journal of Molecular Neuroscience*, 69(3), 263–275.

43. Bellesi, M., et al. (2017). **Sleep and Neuroplasticity.** *Current Biology*, 27(22), R1258–R1260.

44. Delgado, P. L., et al. (2006). **Role of Sleep in Regulating the Brain's Glymphatic System.** *Neuroscience Bulletin*, 22(5), 345–352.

45. Götz, J., et al. (2018). **Role of Tau in Alzheimer's Disease.** *Annual Review of Pathology*, 13, 89–93.

46. Ochsner, K. N., & Gross, J. J. (2005). **The Cognitive Control of Emotion.** *Trends in Cognitive Sciences*, 9(5), 242–249.

47. Brain, T. W., et al. (2016). **The Role of Circadian Rhythms in Cognitive Decline.** *Frontiers in Aging Neuroscience*, 8, 274.

48. Glickman, G., et al. (2006). **Light Therapy and Circadian Rhythms in Cognitive Aging.** *Journal of Biological Rhythms*, 21(2), 108–118.

49. Bredesen, D. E. (2017). The End of Alzheimer's: The First Program to Prevent and Reverse Cognitive Decline. Penguin Publishing.

50. Chen, Z., & Zhong, C. (2013). **Oxidative Stress in Alzheimer's Disease.** *Neuroscience Bulletin*, 30(2), 271–281.

51. Vitetta, L., & Briskey, D. (2015). **Gut Microbiota and Cognitive Decline: How Microbial Metabolites Modulate the Brain.** *Journal of Cellular Biochemistry*, 116(11), 2146–2150.

52. Shokri-Kojori, E., et al. (2018). **Brain Imaging of Alzheimer's Disease: Applications and Innovations**. *Journal of Nuclear Medicine*, 59(6), 786–793.

53. Cummings, J., et al. (2016). **Clinical Trial Endpoints for Alzheimer's Disease Research**. *Alzheimer's & Dementia*, 12(4), 107–117.

54. Wager, T. D., & Atlas, L. Y. (2015). **The Neuroscience of Placebo Effects**. *Nature Reviews Neuroscience*, 16(1), 27–39.

55. Veasey, S. C., et al. (2018). **Circadian Rhythms and Alzheimer's Disease**. *Sleep Medicine Clinics*, 13(3), 383–389.

56. Lucey, B. P., & Holtzman, D. M. (2015). **Sleep and Alzheimer's Disease**. *Brain*, 138(5), 1184–1199.

57. Smith, A. P. (2013). Effects of Nootropics on Cognitive Performance: An Analysis of Clinical Trials. *Nutritional Neuroscience*, 16(5), 206–212.

58. Johnson, D. K., et al. (2018). **The Link Between Physical Activity and Cognitive Decline**. *Journal of Aging Research*, 2018, Article ID 1754195.

59. Kirk, I. J., et al. (2014). **Peptides in Cognitive and Neurodegenerative Diseases**. *Journal of Neurochemistry*, 128(2), 219–227.

60. Whalley, L. J., et al. (2011). **Nootropics and Cognitive Decline: A Meta-Analysis of Controlled Trials**. *Alzheimer's Research & Therapy*, 3(5), 1–12.